# ANXIETY
# C ACH

# ANXIETY COACH

## A Parent's Guide to Treating Childhood Anxiety and OCD

DR. STEPHEN P. H. WHITESIDE

Director of the Mayo Clinic
Pediatric Anxiety Disorders Clinic

MAYO CLINIC PRESS

MAYO CLINIC PRESS
200 First St. SW
Rochester, MN 55905
mcpress.mayoclinic.org



To stay informed about Mayo Clinic Press, please subscribe to our free e-newsletter at mcpress.mayoclinic.org or follow us on social media.

For bulk sales to employers, member groups and health-related companies, contact Mayo Clinic at SpecialSalesMayoBooks@mayo.edu.

Proceeds from the sale of every book benefit important medical research and education at Mayo Clinic.

Cover design: D. Soleil Paz
Cover art: Head Silhouette © Viktoriia_M/Shutterstock.com; Hair © Dedraw Studio/Shutterstock.com

Library of Congress Control Number: 20223036365

ISBN: 979-8-88770-033-5 paperback
ISBN: 979-8-88770-176-9 ebook

Printed in the U.S.A.
First edition: 2024

*To the parents who have trusted me with the care of their children. And the kids and teens who never cease to amaze me with their bravery.*

*To Catherine and Geneva,*
*who make everything possible.*

# Contents

# ANXIETY COACH

# Introduction

For two decades, my colleagues and I, who work with childhood anxiety disorders and obsessive-compulsive disorder (OCD) at Mayo Clinic, in Rochester, Minnesota, have been modifying our pediatric exposure therapy program to be as effective, efficient, and accessible as possible.

We see children and their families from the local community, typically in groups on a once-a-week basis, and also offer a five-day intensive program for kids who don't live within reach of Mayo Clinic or who desire a faster, more concentrated approach. To date, we've worked with thousands of families from all over the U.S. and beyond.

Families often tell us that they value attending our therapy groups because they show them they aren't alone. It might help to know that according to the World Health Organization (WHO), anxiety is the most common psychiatric disorder in the world, with a prevalence of 5.7% to 17.7% in children and adolescents.*

When kids have significant symptoms of anxiety, those symptoms tend to stretch into adolescence and early adulthood, although they may change over time. In younger kids, separation anxiety and specific fears tend to be common. As kids get older and interactions

---

* World Health Organization, "Prevention of Mental Health Disorders: Effective Interventions and Policy Options: Summary Report," 2004, https://www.who.int/publications/i/item/924159215X.

with other kids and friends increase, we start to see higher levels of social anxiety. And as kids reach their teens, their worries may be increasingly about the future and achievement.

Adults with anxiety disorders or OCD often report that their symptoms first began in childhood. Anxiety symptoms can of course be transient and can come and go—a child suffering from anxiety doesn't automatically become an adult suffering from anxiety. But if a child has problems with anxiety, it's a good idea to seek help treating those symptoms to try to make it less likely that they will carry those problems into adulthood.

In addition to the burden of living with excessive fear and worry, over time anxiety disorders can increase the risk of other mental health problems. Kids with anxiety disorders may develop depression, especially when shyness, fears of not being good enough, or worries about making mistakes cause them to miss out on activities that tend to make them happy—sports, activities, clubs, or doing things with friends—and lead to isolation and sadness. This is another reason it's important to treat anxiety disorders in children early, to head off fears and worries before they worsen or lead to other problems.

Our treatment program has two unique aspects. First, we focus almost exclusively on providing exposure therapy: a well-researched intervention designed to help kids face their fears and learn through their own experience that the world is not as scary as their anxiety tells them it is. The second unique aspect of our program is that we work with kids and their parents together the entire time. In these two ways, our approach is very different from more common therapy experiences, in which kids meet with a therapist alone, mostly without their parents present, to learn strategies for coping with anxiety.

In our treatment program, which we call parent-coached exposure therapy, we focus our time in sessions teaching parents how to coach their kids to face their fears. Facing your fears is hard work, and we believe, as a founding principle, that kids will be most successful if they have someone at home to help them work on their anxiety or OCD with exposure therapy. Parents or caregivers are the best people to do that. Kids often go to their parents when they are feeling anxious, and we want parents to feel confident and know how to respond in ways that help their children build confidence.

For a long time, I've wanted to write a guide for parents that shares what we do in our program, in the hope that more kids can benefit from parent-coached exposure therapy. However, I wanted to wait until we could clearly demonstrate that our approach added something new.

In the fall of 2022, we completed a study at Mayo Clinic demonstrating that parent-coached exposure therapy was not only more effective than other therapies for treating anxiety disorders and OCD but that it was also more efficient.

Over one and a half years, we treated 78 kids between the ages of 7 and 17 who had an anxiety disorder or OCD at our anxiety clinic using either our parent-coached exposure therapy or cognitive behavioral therapy (CBT), the most well-researched therapy at the time.

We found that after treatment, the kids who received parent-coached exposure therapy had fewer anxiety symptoms on all measures than the kids who received CBT. And the kids who got parent-coached exposure started to feel better more quickly and ended treatment sooner. It was clear that kids got better faster and with fewer appointments when treatment began with exposures.

I believe you have come to this book because you are seeking understanding and solutions. Watching your child suffer carries its own kind of pain—as a father myself, I can relate. It would be foolish at best and irresponsible at worst for me to make claims that this book can cure your child's anxiety disorder or OCD. Successfully treating anxiety disorders and OCD often requires meeting with a mental health therapist to guide and support you through the process, yet finding a therapist with expertise in childhood anxiety and OCD can be frustratingly hard. Here, I seek to give you the encouragement that what your child is struggling with is very treatable.

The information I've included in this book is the same guidance we give families in our program at Mayo Clinic. The treatment we provide is based on the belief that a parent can learn to be an exposure coach for their child and on a model that has been informed by many years of dedicated clinical expertise and solidified by controlled research.

I am optimistic that this book can set you and your child on the right path to successfully treat their anxiety or OCD. Thank you for giving me the opportunity to share our unique treatment approach with you. My hope for this book is that, after reading it, you will understand childhood anxiety disorders and OCD and their treatment well enough to either tackle exposure therapy with your child at home or be able to make an informed search for an exposure therapist with whom you can work confidently and productively.

# PART 1

## Understanding Anxiety Disorders

In Part 1 of this book we are going to figure out whether the concerns you have about your child are best described as an anxiety disorder, including OCD. Accurately understanding your child's experience is crucial to ensuring that they receive the correct treatment. We're going to start by discussing what separates an anxiety disorder/OCD from normal fears and worries, which we all have, to help you figure out if your child's experience involves feeling more scared or worried than we would expect.

Then, we're going to learn about various anxiety disorder diagnoses, as well as OCD, to see if one or more of the conditions matches your child's experience. We'll then get more specific and explain how to use what we call the avoidance cycle to see if your child's symptoms fit the pattern for how anxiety disorders and OCD work and keep kids stuck.

Finally, we'll learn about other common mental health conditions that may explain your child's symptoms or may need to be addressed before we can begin working on their anxiety or OCD.

My goal is for you to complete Part 1 of this book feeling confident about whether an anxiety disorder or OCD is the best description of what your child is going through and, once you're fairly sure about that, we'll start learning about the best method for treatment: exposure therapy.

It's important to note that reading Part 1 of this book is not sufficient to diagnose your child with an anxiety disorder or OCD. To receive a reliable diagnosis, you need to have your child evaluated by a mental health professional, preferably one with expertise in anxiety disorders and OCD. You can, however, use this section to better understand your child's experience and begin the process of finding them the right help.

# 1

# What Is an Anxiety Disorder?

The first step to helping your child feel better is to make sure you accurately understand their experience. Different mental health conditions require different treatments, which means that getting the right treatment starts by getting the right diagnosis. Within our anxiety disorders program at Mayo Clinic, we start by conducting an assessment to decide whether a child's experience is best described as an anxiety disorder. We approach this as a collaborative process, which may sound unusual since we are the professionals. It's true that the clinicians on our team are experts on anxiety disorders and OCD, but parents are experts on their kids and what they are going through, and, ultimately, kids are the experts on their own lives, feelings, and experiences. Therefore, the goal of the first assessment is to put those areas of expertise together to best understand the child's experience and make the right plan for treatment.

## DEFINING AN ANXIETY DISORDER

A good place for us to start is to make sure we are all on the same page about what an anxiety disorder actually is. Here is how we define an anxiety disorder in our clinic:

**An anxiety disorder involves problems resulting from consistently feeling more nervous, worried, or scared in a situation than would be expected based on a child's abilities.**

We can break this definition down into five parts:

- Feeling nervous, worried, or scared
- More than expected in a situation
- More than expected based on abilities
- Consistently
- Problematic

Let's explore each of these parts in detail, using a fear of dogs as an example. I often use a fear of dogs in our clinic as a working example, because a fear of dogs is both straightforward and easy to picture. Whether kids love dogs or not, they all can visualize a dog and have seen or can imagine someone being afraid of dogs. I love dogs and have had dogs for the past 20 years, yet I was afraid of dogs as a child, so this example really resonates for me in terms of how you can transform fear over time.

To bring this example to life, let's turn to a character, something I'll do throughout this book, as it always helps to have a picture and a story.

Meet 10-year-old Michael. He's been afraid of dogs since he was a little boy. His fear has prevented the family from getting a dog, much to the disappointment of his 13-year-old sister, who loves dogs. His aunt and uncle and other members of the family who have dogs know about his fear and keep their dogs outside or in a kennel when he comes over, which helps. But his fear often prevents him from going to the houses of friends who have dogs, as their families either don't know to be accommodating of his fear or don't have the means to separate the dog from the humans. On top of that, Michael will leave the park straightaway if he sees someone walking their dog and will miss out on playing football with friends. To make matters worse, the neighbor across the street has a large German shepherd that roams around their yard and keeps an eye on the neighborhood. If Michael is playing in his family's front yard when he sees the dog, he runs back inside. He's terrified the German shepherd will bite him or attack him. It's reached the point where he often stays inside the house on the weekends to avoid the neighbor's dog, and he's always keeping an eye out for dogs elsewhere, which means scrutinizing everywhere he goes for the threat of dogs. If he sees a dog while out walking, he panics and crosses the street to avoid it.

With Michael's anxiety in mind, let's look at each of the five parts of our anxiety definition above.

### Feeling nervous, worried, or scared

It may seem obvious that anxiety disorders involve feeling nervous, worried, or scared, but you can't know for sure what a child is feeling inside, so people often make assumptions and sometimes miss the mark. This happens more than you might think, and it turns out that about one-third of the patients we see in our anxiety clinic don't actually have an anxiety disorder. Instead, they have other mental health issues that require different treatments—perhaps for depression or behavior-related issues. That's why goal number one in our clinic, and in this chapter, is to make sure an anxiety disorder is the best understanding of your child's experience.

One reason we see so many kids without anxiety disorders may be that in everyday life we use the term *anxious* to mean different things. Sometimes we say we're anxious when we mean we're feeling nervous or worried. But other times we might talk about being anxious to refer to a more general feeling of distress. And sometimes we might even use *anxious* to mean *excited,* as when we say, *My daughter is really, really, really anxious to see her birthday presents!*

In our clinic and in this book, when talking about anxiety disorders, we are referring to children feeling nervous, worried, or scared, as these are the emotions we experience when we're afraid something bad is going to happen, like someone we care about getting hurt or sick, or Michael fearing a dog will bite him.

These examples and the emotions that go with them are very different from feeling frustrated or angry when we don't get something we believe we deserve, like being passed over for captain of the school swim team or feeling sad or down because we lost someone really important to us, as when a grandparent passes away, or being impatient because we can't wait to do something fun and exciting, like going to the water park.

Feeling anxious encapsulates two separate but related feelings: being scared and being worried. Being scared, or afraid, is an immediate experience, in which we think that something bad is about to happen right here, right now. This is how we might feel when we stand up to give a presentation in front of the class or when an unfamiliar large dog barks and charges at us.

Worry, on the other hand, is anxiety about something that might happen in the future or possibly happened in the past. This might include worrying that you will fail an upcoming test and never get a good job or worrying that you said something wrong at school yesterday and everyone is talking about you. There are important differences between immediate fear and future worry, including the parts of the brain involved; what combines them is that they both involve feeling nervous that something bad will happen.

Being afraid, worried, or nervous is normal and an important part of being human. If you never felt afraid, worried, or nervous, that would be a problem because these feelings help keep us safe.

Does that mean anxiety can actually be good for us? In short, yes. Anxiety, fear, nervousness, and worry are essential and serve as safety tools and, in the face of potential danger, alarm bells. We need these feelings to survive. They help us stay safe and do things now to prepare for the future.

Anxiety reminds us to look both ways when we cross the street. It helps us decide not to do things that may be dangerous. It helps us leave situations where we can potentially be hurt. Worrying about not doing well at school motivates your child to study hard, check their answers, and turn their homework in on time.

Worrying that your child is going to have a bad day if they don't get enough sleep or have a good breakfast helps you as a parent make the decision to get the kids to bed on time or run to the grocery store, even if it would be more fun to stay up and hang out with them a little bit more. Worrying three months before our summer vacation that it won't be very fun if we don't have enough activities planned for the trip and coming up with extra ideas in advance is adaptive and will likely lead to a more fulfilling vacation. That worry is helpful and creates healthy family routines.

In the same way, feeling nervous when you see a dog growling, and thinking, *You know what, I'm going to avoid this dog,* is a smart move because you're paying attention to signs alerting you that this dog may not be friendly. That nervousness may save you from getting jumped on, scratched, or bitten. Fear, nervousness, and worry are therefore adaptive and practical and central to healthy living and everyday safety.

Anxiety motivates us to take action by activating our sympathetic nervous system, which revs up the body to protect us by making our heartbeat and breathing faster and releasing adrenaline that can result in making us hyperalert and full of energy. This is called the fight or flight response, and it's a valuable mechanism if you are actually in danger. If you go on a family camping trip and wake in the night to hear a noise in the woods that may be the sound of a wild animal, your attention needs to be sharply focused for any sign of movement, and your body needs to be ready to physically protect your family. There is also a third response to danger, which is freezing, in which we stay perfectly still in the hope that if there is something out there, it won't see us and will move on.

Although the fight or flight response is helpful, even essential, when faced with physical danger, it is less helpful in many modern-day situations that cause anxiety, like giving a presentation in class, worrying about your grade on a test, or separating from parents before school. In these situations, the fight or flight (or freezing) response can make a child feel worse: embarrassed by how sweaty they are, unable to shift attention from thoughts of worry, clamming up and shutting down, or feeling sick to their stomach.

If anxiety and feeling nervous, worried, or scared is normal and necessary, albeit sometimes inconvenient, what makes it a problem? The answer to that question brings us to the next part of what makes up an anxiety disorder.

### More than expected in a situation

An anxiety disorder involves a child being more nervous in a situation than most other kids would be. If 99 kids find making a presentation to their class unpleasant but they know they can do it, and one kid can't sleep for a week before the presentation, begs to get out of it, and stays home from school the day of the presentation with a stomachache, that one kid likely has an anxiety disorder.

Let's go back to Michael and his neighbor's German shepherd. The dog loves people, and almost everybody in the neighborhood knows and loves this dog. However, this dog gets excited and barks a lot if she feels she is not getting enough attention. If Michael is afraid of that dog when every other kid on the street likes her and thinks she's cute, then he may have an anxiety disorder; he is afraid of something that is generally, by social consensus, considered safe, and that other kids in the neighborhood are not afraid of.

On the other hand, let's say there's another neighbor with a dog, and this dog is poorly trained, generally mean, and everyone on the street knows that it once bit the mail carrier. They feel that, given that background, it really ought to be kept behind the fence. Most people who live on this street make sure to stay away from this dog and feel nervous passing by when it aggressively barks at them from the front yard. If Michael is afraid of *this* dog but not of the German shepherd, his fear is not a sign of an anxiety disorder. Instead, he's reacting to a stressful situation. He still feels nervous, worried, or scared, but so do other adults and kids who live on the street when they encounter this dog.

Differentiating between whether a child has an anxiety disorder or is responding to a stressful situation is one of the main things that needs to be established before beginning treatment. If a child has an anxiety disorder, we have to help them face their fears and to learn through their own experience that the thing they're afraid of is not actually dangerous.

If instead the child is experiencing anxiety due to a stressful situation, then we need to help fix the cause of the stress or avoid the situation altogether, like all residents on the street joining forces to petition the neighbor with the mean dog to keep the dog leashed, fenced, or supervised when it's on the front lawn and visible to passersby.

Another example would be a child worrying about the possible death of a parent who is fit and healthy—this may be an anxiety disorder—versus a child who is worrying about the death of a parent who has recently been diagnosed with cancer. The latter is a perfectly natural response—most kids would be worried about a sick parent, and therefore their anxiety is not a symptom or sign of a psychological disorder. Conversely, very few children will spend their time worrying about a parent who is fit and healthy, so in that child's case, the signs point to an anxiety disorder.

Similarly, a teenager worrying about not getting into college if she doesn't get straight As—even though she mostly does get straight As—likely has an anxiety disorder, while a teenager worrying about not graduating from high school because she is currently failing many of her classes is in a problematic situation, and feeling worried is not only entirely legitimate but also appropriate.

In the case of the student failing her classes, the problem lies with what has led to her failing classes. Maybe she is skipping classes, not spending enough time doing her homework, or not adequately studying for tests. The remedy for her worry would be to address the problems that led to her bad grades—she could get help with her study skills, with structuring time to ensure her homework is completed, or with ensuring she attends class. Treatment obviously should not focus on convincing her to worry less about failing school. This contrasts with the teenager described above who generally gets straight As and whose anxiety is out of sync with the reality of her academic success and whose treatment needs to focus on helping her worry less.

In a final example, a child who doesn't want to go to school because he feels too nervous to talk to people, even though his peers generally like him and the school day is uneventful, might have an anxiety disorder. However, if he is too nervous to go to school and talk to peers because he is being teased and bullied, he does not have a problem with anxiety; rather, he is in a very stressful situation that requires an intervention by his parents or teachers or a school counselor to stop the mistreatment.

You might be thinking at this point that every child is different, and just because some kids can handle a situation doesn't mean that all kids can. And this brings us to the third part of how we understand what constitutes an anxiety disorder.

### More than expected based on abilities

We just talked about how an anxiety disorder differs from feeling nervous, worried, or scared in situations that most people would find generally stressful. However, not all kids find the same situations stressful, so we also have to pay attention to a child's abilities when separating anxiety disorders from stressful circumstances.

If a child or teenager is asked to do something they know they can't do, they will likely get nervous about doing it. Not because they have a problem with being overly anxious but because they accurately know that the situation probably won't turn out well. For example, being nervous about the prospect of staying home alone for 30 minutes after school would suggest an anxiety disorder if the child is 14 years old but would not be particularly surprising if the child is 5 years old. Societally speaking, we expect most 14-year-olds to have the capability to take care of themselves alone at home, whereas we do not have a collective expectation that most 5-year-olds can do so.

If we return to the example of worrying about grades, the teen who gets very nervous before a test, but generally gets straight As, may have an anxiety disorder because she is overly nervous despite being very capable. But if a child is failing classes because they don't understand their assignments, can't stay focused in class, and lose their homework, their worry about failing is not an anxiety disorder, it's a perfectly normal and very healthy reaction to consistent academic struggles. The real problem here may be that this child's learning needs are not being met, and we would likely want to evaluate the child for attention deficit hyperactivity disorder (ADHD) because they can't keep track of their assignments or hold focus long enough to get them done. Or maybe they have an undiagnosed learning disability and reading is more difficult for them than for their peers and that's why they're struggling to complete assignments. In this case, it would make no sense to help that child be less nervous about the prospect of failing school because that is a real possibility; instead, they need help to be successful.

Feeling anxious about social situations provides another example of why it's important to understand a child's abilities. Some children have social skill deficits and struggle with interacting or understanding what other kids are thinking or feeling. They may have trouble reading social situations and just as much trouble relating to what other kids are interested in, so when they try to talk to other kids it doesn't go as well as they hoped, because other kids tend to get uncomfortable and walk away. As unsuccessful social interactions compound, this child may understandably become anxious about social situations. But the problem here is not their anxiety, it's that they don't yet have the skills to be successful socially. In that scenario, a counselor might be needed to help the child develop their ability to start conversations and build other social skills.

When deciding whether a child is feeling more nervous about a scenario than we would typically expect, it's important to pay attention to the situation they are in as well as their own skills and ability to be successful in that situation. We also have to

When deciding whether a child is feeling more nervous about a scenario than we would typically expect, it's important to pay attention to the situation they are in as well as their own skills and ability to be successful in that situation.

pay attention to how often it happens, which brings us to the fourth part of what makes up an anxiety disorder.

## Consistently

When a child has an anxiety disorder, they will almost always feel nervous in their feared situations. A child who fears being away from parents typically gets upset every morning before going to school. But if some days this child separates from her parents before school just fine with no apparent anxiety and on other days she becomes demonstrably upset, this suggests a different problem. Maybe she isn't nervous about separation, but instead there's something else going on at school that particular day that makes her nervous, like gym class, because she is a slow runner and her classmates keep teasing her about it. Or maybe it has nothing to do with school and instead she's just not much of a morning person, and there are days where she was doing homework late and reading in bed even later so that she didn't get enough sleep, and now she's cranky and drags her feet about going to school, which comes off like she's nervous about separating.

By *consistently* we don't mean that a child is afraid of every related situation that we could expect them to be nervous about. Children who are very nervous in social situations, such as meeting new people and talking in class, will often have a handful of close friends with whom they feel totally comfortable. In this case, a child still has significant social anxiety, because they always feel nervous meeting new people.

Similarly, parents sometimes ask me why their teenager, who constantly washes his hands because of fears of germs making him sick, leaves his room in a continuously messy state. They have a point. Here's a teenager whose bedroom looks like a tornado blew through it but who covers his hand with his sleeve to push a door open in public and who uses hand sanitizer every time he touches a desk, chair, textbook, menu, and more. This teen still has OCD because he consistently fears germs in public places, even though he doesn't fear his room being in disarray. (We'll be looking at OCD in a lot more detail later, so don't worry if this doesn't totally make sense at this stage.)

The concept of consistency is often difficult to apply, since kids' fears can be very specific and may not occur in all the situations parents expect them to, especially if we don't fully understand those fears yet. Returning to the fear of dogs example, if Michael is always afraid of dogs even when there is every reason to believe they are perfectly harmless, that sounds a lot like an anxiety disorder. If he is always afraid of large dogs but not small dogs, this also suggests an anxiety disorder. If he has no problem with Grandma and Grandpa's large and loud German shepherd, Jessie, whom he has known his whole life, but he is very afraid of every other dog he encounters, then we would still likely be looking at an anxiety disorder. However, if he is usually fine around all dogs including the neighbor's dog but sporadically gets very upset when the neighbor's dog is outside in the front yard, then it starts to seem a lot less likely that he has an anxiety disorder.

Another rule of thumb with consistency is that the anxiety happens regularly over an extended period of time. Having one frightened reaction or a period of intermittent frightened reactions does not necessarily point to an anxiety disorder. An anxiety disorder is persistent. That doesn't mean that we should wait for a child's anxiety to become really severe. It means that if a child's problems with anxiety come and go over time, we don't necessarily have to jump in and work on it, which brings us to the fifth and final part of how we think about anxiety disorders.

## Problematic

An important aspect of how we understand anxiety disorders is that they are a problem. And this is important because, if anxiety is not a problem, then we don't necessarily need to do anything about it. I define *problem* here as anxiety getting in the way of everyday life and making it hard for your child to do the things they need and want to do, which, in turn, affects you as well.

By contrast, if a child's experience meets all parts of our definition, and he is consistently more nervous about a scenario than we would expect him to be, but it doesn't upset him or stop him from doing the things he needs and wants to do, then there may be no reason to seek out additional support or pursue treatment.

Earlier, we talked about how anxiety is not only normal but a protecting, cautionary, and essential part of our human makeup and experience. We all know that each child is unique. Some are tall, some are short. Some like to run around and be active, others would rather sit and read a good book. This same variation applies to anxiety as well. Some kids worry about whether things will turn out okay, while others tend to assume everything will be just fine. Some children are outgoing and love meeting new people, others are shy and prefer spending time with close friends and family. Some kids can't wait to get away from their parents for a new adventure, others prefer to stick close to their parents, siblings, and the comforts of home. All of this variation is entirely normal. The human population is diverse, and this keeps life interesting.

As part of this variation, there is nothing necessarily wrong with your child being shy, a worrier, or a nervous, cautious person. I recall a mom of two daughters saying that one daughter was incredibly sociable, had a lot of friends, and had a busy social calendar, and the other daughter was shy, stayed home a lot, and had a small group of friends. The mom, who was very sociable herself, was worried about the shy daughter and wondered if she should arrange a mental health assessment. But both daughters were happy, successful at school, and had friends they liked to be with. There was no problem here; the mom simply had one sociable daughter and one shy daughter. Differences are just that: differences.

As another example, when I ask kids who come to the clinic if they have any big fears, spiders often come up. They'll say something like, *I'm really scared of spiders. Whenever I see a spider, I run out of the room screaming.* To this, they often also add a line like, *Even though I'm freaking out, I usually go back into the room and kill the spider myself.* Talking it over, we realize that we don't actually need to do any work on their fear of spiders, because this fear isn't causing any disruption to their everyday life. And when push comes to shove, they are capable of grabbing a shoe and disposing of the spider. (Not that I have anything against spiders or encourage their demise.)

So, as a parent, how do you ultimately know if your child's anxiety has become a problem? There are two key questions to consider: One, does the anxiety stop your child from doing things they need and want to do? And two, is the anxiety upsetting them in a visible way?

As I see it, children have three jobs: school, friends, and family. To be successful academically, kids should be going to school and getting their work done. They don't have to be getting straight As to be considered successful, but they do need to be putting forth a good effort. To be successful socially, kids should have at least two or three close friends they hang out with informally outside of school and also take part in fun activities, whether structured extracurriculars like sports, dance, and clubs or informal hobbies. And finally, kids should be interacting at home with their family and helping out with chores around the house.

How all three roles look in reality will vary greatly from family to family, child to child, school to school, age to age, et cetera. But generally speaking, we can use these as a benchmark to measure whether kids are on track.

One way to determine if your child may have an anxiety disorder is to consider whether anxiety is getting in the way of one or more of these jobs. If your child is really interested in soccer or ballet but so nervous about being around new kids that they won't sign up for the activity, that's a red flag. Or if they do sign up, but when it's time to attend the first class they get upset and refuse to leave the house, again, a red flag. If over time, rather than doing fun activities, they sit at home, where they get bored and feel sad because they're left out of activities that other kids are doing and that they want to do too, but don't feel like they can, that points to an anxiety disorder.

Anxiety can also sometimes get in the way of kids doing things that their parents need them to do. For example, a child who fears separating from her parents might refuse to stay with a sitter or relatives who live nearby, so now her parents have to forgo their date night.

The other way that anxiety can be a problem is that even if your child is doing what they need to do, anxiety makes those activities challenging and upsetting. Maybe your son is really nervous about being around other kids because he fears he will say the wrong thing or make a mistake. Despite this anxiety, he still goes to school, has a couple close friends, and plays on the basketball team. On the weekend, despite his fears, he finds time to go to extra basketball practice with the team and also helps his dad mow the lawn and tidy the yard. In other words, he's competently doing all three of his jobs.

However, looking closer, there's no mistaking he's miserable. Mornings before school are tough for the family because he often complains of stomachaches and doesn't want to go. He will also skip basketball practice when he knows his one friend on the team is out with the flu. At night, falling asleep is hard, because he can't stop thinking about the social situations that happened during the day. He replays conversations and encounters over and over in his head, trying to spot if he said anything embarrassing. In this case, despite him fulfilling his three jobs, social anxiety is making life harder and more upsetting for him than it needs to be, even though it's not stopping him from doing what he needs to. He likely has an anxiety disorder even though he is heroically trying to keep up with everything expected of him.

Kids going through anxiety can be high-achieving and doing all the things they're supposed to be doing. They're getting good grades. They're involved in an activity. They have close friends. But they are also really upset on the inside and avoid a lot of situations. This could look like going to school without resistance but once there, avoiding talking to other kids. They have the same couple of friends they've had for a long time, but even that clique has been dwindling because kids' interests change and they haven't been able to make new friends because they're too nervous to branch out. If this sounds like your child, you may find it harder to notice the incremental drift toward anxiety having more and more power over your child's life.

---

I hope this information has increased your confidence to know whether your child's experience is best described as an anxiety disorder. As a parent, you are the expert on your child, and you know your child better than any mental health professional ever will. Of course, and very appropriately, you're not expected to know everything about your child and how he or she feels, especially as children turn into teenagers and seek more independence.

In the next chapter we'll get more specific by going over the different anxiety disorders to see which one or ones best describe your child's experience. As a side note, let me say at this time that it's quite okay if you are still not entirely sure whether your child has an anxiety disorder. Sometimes going through the list of specific disorders helps crystallize understanding of whether or not your child's experience fits into the overall anxiety disorders category.

# 2

# What Are the Different Anxiety Disorders?

There are various anxiety disorders that may describe your child's experience. Even though we treat all anxiety disorders and OCD with exposure therapy, the specific activities we do during treatment differ for each diagnosis. Therefore, once we have decided that a child's experience fits our definition of an anxiety disorder, it is helpful to next focus more specifically on which anxiety disorder diagnosis provides the best fit. This puts us one step closer to making a treatment plan tailored to your child's needs. In the final section of this book, you'll find a series of chapters dedicated to applying methods of exposure therapy to each specific anxiety disorder.

## WHAT ARE MENTAL HEALTH DIAGNOSES?

Before we get into specific anxiety diagnoses, it might help to talk a little about what a mental health diagnosis actually means. In our clinic, I explain that mental health diagnoses are ways of describing how kids think, feel, and act. They are not names of diseases. There is nothing broken per se or not working correctly in the body that we can test or measure the way doctors can for kidney disease, type 1 diabetes, a wrist fracture, or a heart condition.

Parents who contact our clinic have sometimes heard about chemical imbalances in the brain and will ask if we do any medical tests or brain scans to accurately arrive at a diagnosis. While research is ever evolving, there are currently no blood or imaging tests that can be used to diagnose anxiety disorders or other mental health conditions.

If we don't use medical tests to diagnose anxiety disorders, what do we do? Mental health disorders are descriptions of ways in which children think, feel, and act and how their behaviors or thoughts can manifest as a problem. There are two sources for these descriptions and diagnoses, one published by the American Psychiatric Association and the other by the World Health Organization. Both are pretty similar. When we talk about mental health in the U.S., we typically use the diagnostic system from the American Psychiatric Association, called the Diagnostic and Statistical Manual, known as the DSM-5 for short.

The DSM-5 lists all mental health disorders and the symptoms that have to be present for each to warrant a formal diagnosis. Diagnosing a child with a mental health disorder should involve meeting with a mental health professional, talking through your concerns, answering specific questions related to any relevant conditions, and then the mental health professional deciding whether or not your child has all the symptoms needed to meet the criteria for a diagnosis.

A mental health professional needs to gather information from both the child and parents or other caregivers to get a full, comprehensive portrait of symptoms. I think it is beneficial for parents to feel like they are working with the mental health professional, rather than simply being told what the mental health professional believes is going on with their child. My goal when diagnosing a child with an anxiety disorder is that the child, their parents, and our team are all in agreement that the diagnosis is accurate.

I want parents to feel they can tell me if I didn't understand something correctly or if I am getting stuck on something that is not nearly as important to them as something else I am missing. Without this shared agreement, it is unlikely that families will find the assessment helpful or informative.

Although we don't use blood tests or imaging in the diagnostic process, we often use assessment questionnaires. Mental health questionnaires generally ask kids and parents to rate how often the child has a feeling, thought, or behavior. The responses are then added up to give a score for how severe the child's symptoms are. Questionnaires can be helpful in putting a number on the severity of a child's symptoms, which can then be useful for deciding how much of a problem the child's symptoms are compared to the experiences of other kids and for tracking progress over time. Questionnaires are a quick and convenient way to make sure we gather as much accurate information as possible from the child and parents concerning symptoms.

With this in mind, let's now have a quick introduction to the individual anxiety disorders.

## THE ANXIETY DISORDERS

### Social anxiety disorder

The term *social anxiety disorder* fits when children are overly nervous about interacting with other people, particularly peers. Kids with social anxiety are afraid they will make mistakes when talking or will say or do something that could lead other people to think of them negatively. Feeling nervous leads kids to avoid situations that involve talking with or hanging out with or even being around other kids. When children with social anxiety disorder consistently avoid social situations, it means they miss out on fun activities, like sports, or don't do things they need to do, like give a class presentation. Over time, missing out on these important activities can cause other problems. Social anxiety disorder is one of the most common reasons families come to our clinic.

> Social anxiety disorder is different from typical shyness in the degree of anxiety that kids experience and how much their fears cause problems.

Social anxiety disorder is different from typical shyness in the degree of anxiety that kids experience and how much their fears cause problems. There is nothing wrong with being shy or introverted; I myself was pretty shy as a child. Being nervous giving presentations at school or starting a new activity is also a very normal, common experience. As I mentioned earlier, it's important not to unnecessarily label your child's behavior as a problem. If they are content with the way they are living their life and they are doing the school and social activities they need to, that's a solid sign that all is well.

However, when fears of embarrassment are so upsetting that they get in the way of living everyday life, that's when we call it social anxiety disorder and recommend treatment. There are times in our clinic when kids and parents disagree on whether social anxiety is a problem. This usually happens in two scenarios. Since many social interactions for kids occur in school, without parents there to witness their child's difficulties, parents have only the impression they get from seeing their child function in the family setting, whether that's at home or in public. In these cases, parents may not realize how much their teens or kids are struggling socially. Other times, it's the reverse, and kids are so upset by their social difficulties that they deny they are nervous and instead say they are simply not interested in spending time with other kids, and what is wrong with that conscious choice, if they are making it? In that and similar kinds of cases, we need to focus on the three jobs we expect from kids and teens—being successful in school, with friends, and at home—and if there are problems in those areas, we can explore how social anxiety might be getting in the way.

To illustrate social anxiety, let's look at 16-year-old Maria, a smart, likable teenager and a successful figure skater. She and her parents agreed that she had always been shy, but it hadn't been a problem because she'd maintained a core group of friends since kindergarten. In restaurants, she'd appear nervous, and her parents would order for her, but they weren't overly concerned about it. None of this was a problem until she entered middle school. With that transition, she began to struggle. Her core friends connected with new faces and added new friends, while Maria stayed on the sidelines, feeling shy. She felt even more nervous in class when she didn't yet know many of the other students and, with seven different classes a day, there wasn't much of a chance to get to know her teachers. In this new environment, she came to dread presentations, yet was too nervous to ask for help. Under pressure across the board, some of her grades began to slip. When Maria began to complain that she felt too sick to go to school on days she had a class where there was always a lot of student participation, her parents brought her in for help.

During the initial assessment, Maria readily acknowledged that in social situations she was afraid she would say the wrong thing and look ridiculous in front of other kids who all seemed to be calm, outgoing, and happy to make new friends and expand their social circle. She had always felt comfortable with figure skating because so much of it involved working on her own without having to make conversation with the other skaters. However, now that they were getting older and spending more time chitchatting before and after practice, she was struggling with these interactions and feeling awkward. It had reached a point where she felt left out and was considering quitting.

After a diagnosis of social anxiety disorder was agreed upon, Maria signed up to start treatment with exposure therapy.

### Generalized anxiety disorder

Generalized anxiety disorder (GAD) describes the tendency to worry and be nervous about a lot of different things a lot of the time. Kids with GAD tend to worry about doing well at sports or school, getting into trouble, their health and personal safety, the health and safety of their family, people breaking into the family home, getting into a car accident, or never getting a good job when they grow up. In other words, just about everything. They sometimes worry that they are worrying too much.

As with social anxiety, let's be clear: There is nothing wrong with worrying about things. If your child is totally unprepared for the math test they have tomorrow, worrying about failing will hopefully motivate them to go all out in studying the evening before.

What distinguishes and makes GAD worries problematic is that kids are worrying about situations that have no warning signs, will likely turn out fine, and have little to no chance of happening. They worry about getting into college even though they get straight As, they worry about their parents' health even though both parents are fit and healthy, they worry about a burglar coming in their bedroom window at night even though they live in a safe neighborhood with no reports of burglary.

What distinguishes and makes GAD worries problematic is that kids are worrying about situations that have no warning signs, will likely turn out fine, and have little to no chance of happening.

Worrying more than others does not automatically mean that we need to call it a disorder. As we discussed earlier, worrying helps us all to be responsible and take care of ourselves and others and to make sure things turn out safely and successfully. If some kids worry too much and are a little too responsible or caring or hardworking, that really isn't a problem. There's a reason we have expressions like "better safe than sorry" and "better to err on the side of caution."

What's key here is that worrying enters the realm of GAD when it is upsetting to your child and causes problems in their everyday life. For it to reach this level, worrying will be taking up a lot of their time—worrying most days of the week, week in and week out. At a GAD level it is hard for the child to stop worrying. If a child tends to get nervous about many things but can get back in control and easily and independently push the worries away, he or she probably isn't experiencing GAD.

Another part of GAD is that all this worrying starts to affect how kids and teens are feeling physically. Kids with GAD often feel tired and have trouble sleeping. They feel tense and irritable, have headaches or stomachaches, and find it hard to concentrate. Every child feels these ways at times, but kids with GAD feel this way often, especially when they are worried.

To bring GAD to life, let's talk about 14-year-old Kara, a high-achieving girl who came for an evaluation with her parents because she was stressed out about everything. Her parents were particularly concerned that she was not getting enough sleep, which led her to be irritable with her family. Kara responded that there wasn't anything she could do about it because she had to get her homework done, which sometimes took until midnight. Despite being a straight-A student, one of Kara's primary worries was not doing well enough at school. She was constantly frightened of disappointing people and terrified that she would mess up and harm her grades enough to prevent her from going to college and eventually securing a good job. These worries led her to spend much more time completing homework than needed, even though it was clear that Kara could be successful at school with moderate effort. But she went far beyond this and typically checked her assignments multiple times, shot past the required length for writing assignments, completed extra-credit tasks, and studied excessively for tests. This amount of extra work left little time for socializing, sleep, or activities she enjoyed, like watching movies and meeting friends for bubble tea.

Although fear of academic failure was her most prominent symptom, Kara had a wide variety of worries surrounding getting in trouble (despite always following the rules), the family's finances (despite no hint of problems or parental concern), and the health of her parents and siblings (despite all of them being fit and healthy). After some assurance that the goal of exposure therapy was not to make her get bad grades but instead to help her manage her fears around getting bad grades without staying up all night, Kara acknowledged that she would like to feel less stressed out all the time and agreed to give treatment a try.

### Separation anxiety disorder

With separation anxiety disorder, young children and sometimes older children and teenagers feel very nervous or afraid of being separated from their parents, even for a short period of time.

With separation anxiety disorder, young children and sometimes older children and teenagers feel very nervous or afraid of being separated from their parents, even for a short period of time.

What is common or expected for separation has a lot to do with the child's age. Anxiety when first going to preschool or kindergarten is not unusual. Similarly, older kids might feel nervous going off to sleepaway camp for the first time or when a parent leaves for a weeklong work trip. In these situations, anxiety around separation is generally short-lived and goes away as the child gets used to school or camp or the parent returns home. For some kids, their fears and worries don't improve and may even get worse. Tearful goodbyes with multiple hugs turn into screaming, clinging, or refusing to get out of the car. Complaints about upset stomachs and not wanting to go to school begin the night before and continue into the morning.

When kids are experiencing separation anxiety disorder they often worry that something bad will happen to them or their parents while they are separated, such as their being kidnapped or their parents leaving for a work event and never coming back because they get into a car accident. Other times, especially with younger children, even though they are very upset to be separated from their parents, they may not be able to articulate their worries. Then there are some kids who are too nervous to be left in a room alone and follow their parents around the house, from room to room, becoming very upset when a parent disappears for a few minutes to use the bathroom.

Bedtime can be a stressful time for families whose child has separation anxiety disorder. A kid feeling too nervous to be alone in their bedroom may repeatedly cry out or keep coming out of their room until a parent returns to comfort them. In desperation, parents often begin to lie down with their child until the child falls asleep, or even routinely let the child sleep in their bed. Needless to say, this can become exhausting over time. Co-sleeping is not a problem if it is consistent with the family's preferences or expectations. However, when anxiety, fear, tears, and clinging routinely interfere with going to school, a simple bedtime transition, or staying home with a sitter, this is likely to be separation anxiety disorder.

Eight-year-old Alex never slept on his own and because his mother frequently dozed off while waiting for him to fall asleep, she had fallen into a long-term habit of sleeping in his bed. His parents had not been out at night without the children for as long as they could remember. They gave up because Alex would cry and cling to them whenever they tried to leave him, and, if they actually made it out for an evening by leaving him with his grandparents—the only people he would even consider being left alone with—he'd make his grandmother call his parents repeatedly to check how long until they'd be home.

Going to school had not been a problem because his mother worked at the school as an assistant in the office. A few times a week he would become tearful in class and ask permission to go to the school office to see his mother, where she would comfort him. Alex's parents decided it was time to seek help after his mother got a new job at another school and dropping him off in the morning at his school became challenging. The disruption continued until Alex built his confidence to be independent through exposure therapy.

### Specific phobia

Whereas kids with GAD worry about many different topics, kids with specific phobias have one intense fear, such as of the dark, bees, or heights. Although kids can certainly have more than one phobia—for example, they may be afraid of bees and storms—the gist of a specific phobia is that a child's fear is typically focused on a single theme.

The possible themes that can be the subject of a kid's fears are as broad as the world and everything within it, but the common fears that we see in our clinic include the dark, needles, shots, blood draws, vomiting, storms, bugs, bees, wasps, spiders, and heights. We also see less common fears such as buttons, bread, mascots, and even small intricate patterns. Due to the wide variety of themes that can arouse fear, phobias are organized into five categories: animals, natural environments (like the dark or storms), blood-injection-injury (like needles or seeing blood), situational (like elevators), and other (where we would put a fear of vomiting or loud sounds).

As with all anxiety disorders, these fears need to be in excess of the situation, lead to avoidance, and have reached a stage of being problematic and life-disrupting. Most kids find shots unpleasant, if not scary or painful, but are able to grimace through receiving recommended vaccines and other medical care with a bit of supportive coaching from a parent or nurse. On the other hand, some kids become so afraid of getting shots that they shake and cry and have to be helped by multiple nurses to get their needed shots or they may even faint at the sight of a needle, experiences that make their fears grow even bigger for the next time. For these kids, even though their fear of needles doesn't come up that often—most kids don't need shots too frequently—it causes real problems when it does. Sometimes, the fear of shots expands to doctors in general, so kids become afraid of any medical appointment in case it may involve getting a shot or having blood drawn, even if their parents assure them to the contrary.

Other specific phobias affect kids on a day-to-day basis. A lot of children find storms nerve-racking, but for some, they are terrifying. They fear that a tornado will blow in and destroy their home or a lightning bolt will strike the roof and set the house on fire. Kids with these phobias tend to become very upset during storms. Not only that, they may also worry there will be a really bad storm whenever it's cloudy or overcast and constantly check the weather report to see if a storm is predicted. Even if there is no storm, the mere sight of gray skies may be enough to set their nerves on edge.

Eight-year-old Aaron had an intense fear of heights. His fear came up most frequently around slides and jungle gyms at the park, where he would feel too nervous to climb or swing. He also became very concerned when his younger brother wanted to run off and play at the park. His fears extended to elevators and escalators as well, which led the family to often take the stairs or resulted in Aaron closing his eyes and clinging to his mother when elevators were the only option. In addition to his fear of heights beginning to interfere with friendships due to his anxiety on the playground, after a vacation during which Aaron's refusal to take elevators made their stay in a room on the 12th floor of a hotel impossible, his parents decided to seek help.

### Panic disorder and agoraphobia

Whereas kids with a specific phobia have a clear, definable fear, kids with panic disorder become suddenly frightened for no clear reason at all. Panic attacks are very sudden episodes of fear and anxiety during which kids experience intense physical symptoms such as feeling like their heart is pounding, having difficulty breathing, feeling like their surroundings are spinning, shaking legs or hands, breaking into a cold sweat, getting dizzy, or getting nauseous.

It's not uncommon for children or teenagers to have panic attacks, particularly in stressful situations, like having to talk in front of the class at school. However, with panic disorder, the panic attacks seem to happen for no reason when the child is not in a feared situation or overly worried. Panic attacks, especially when they come out of nowhere, can be very frightening.

It's not uncommon for children or teenagers to have panic attacks, particularly in stressful situations, like having to talk in front of the class at school. However, with panic disorder, the panic attacks seem to happen for no reason when the child is not in a feared situation or overly worried.

After experiencing a panic attack, kids may become fearful of having another, especially of having one at an inconvenient time, like in school or all by themselves without their parents there to help. At that point, kids can also develop agoraphobia, in which they are scared to go out in public due to fear that if they have a panic attack or feel anxious it will be hard to leave or get help. Both panic disorder and agoraphobia are less common in kids than the other anxiety disorders we have discussed.

Thirteen-year-old Nora was afraid to go to school. When her parents took her to see a mental health professional, she couldn't explain why. She was not nervous to talk to people, generally felt comfortable with kids at school, had a group of good friends, and was not being teased or bullied. On top of this, she was a good student, receiving mostly Bs, and could probably do better if she put in more consistent effort. She thought her teachers were good, and so were her classes. However, over the past few months she had become so anxious in school that she asked permission to leave class and go to the bathroom, where she'd call her parents to pick her up. When she did this, she'd say her heart was pounding, she couldn't catch her breath, and she was shaking and sweating. Not only was this experience frightening, but she was convinced that everyone in class could tell what was happening to her, and she was terrified that she would lose control and start crying right there in class. These episodes were so upsetting that she started to dread going to school and was having more and more difficulty leaving the house in the morning. Nora also described smaller episodes taking place at home, which were less upsetting for her, because there was no audience beyond her parents and younger sister, and she could go to her room and be alone until the attack passed. However, after experiencing a panic attack while out shopping, she no longer felt comfortable going to stores and preferred to stay home. That was the tipping point that led her parents to seek out professional help, where they were introduced to panic disorder and agoraphobia as well as their treatment through exposure therapy.

### Obsessive compulsive disorder

Obsessive compulsive disorder (OCD) is a mental health disorder that involves two sets of symptoms. First, children have obsessions, which are scary or upsetting thoughts that happen over and over again. These are also called intrusive thoughts because they are unwanted and appear to intrude on a child's thinking. For example, kids with OCD might repeatedly think they have germs on their hands that might make them sick or have the thought that something bad is going to happen or that they will do something bad. These thoughts are very upsetting because the child does not want to get sick or have bad things happen, and having the thoughts makes them afraid that either may occur. To manage this, the child does something to feel better or safer and this is the second symptom: compulsions. Kids might wash their hands or use hand sanitizer many times a day, every time they fear they've come into contact with germs. They might lock and unlock and relock the front door or turn a light switch off and on and off again until they feel sure they did it right. Or they might walk back and forth through a doorway multiple times until they can do it with a safe thought instead of an intrusive, scary thought. Or they might ask their parents over and over if they are in trouble for some reason or repeatedly apologize for something trivial and unimportant or for something that didn't actually happen. Kids complete these repetitive actions because these compulsions relieve the anxiety from their obsessive thoughts.

A child with OCD might have an intrusive thought like, *If I walk through the door while I'm having a thought about cancer I'm going to get cancer.* This thought feels overwhelming, and even if they know it is unlikely to come true, it feels safest to fix it. So, to relieve their anxiety, they walk back out and then pass through the door again with a replacement thought, something like, *I'm a healthy person.* Unfortunately, sometimes the child might not be able to fully get the first thought out of their head, which leads to walking back and forth through the door repeatedly until they feel satisfied that they have undone the first thought.

For a child's experience to be diagnosed as OCD, their symptoms need to be problematic. Many people like to have things a certain way or double-check things unnecessarily. At my house we have a light in the stairwell that can be turned on and off by either a light switch at the bottom of the stairs or one at the top of stairs. The lights are off when the switches are both up or both down, it doesn't matter which. I, however, think it is best to turn the lights off by having both switches pointed down in the traditional off position. So, I will sometimes walk up the stairs in the dark, rather than turning them on downstairs and then off when I get upstairs because this would leave them in the "wrong" up position. Silly, isn't it? The lights are just as off and the stairs are just as dark if both switches are up or down. One way simply feels right to me. But that is not OCD, because I can leave them in the wrong position and move on just fine. When someone has OCD, when something feels wrong, they believe they can't just move on. They have to repeat the action and check it until they get it right, even though they would rather not, even though it is taking way too much time.

OCD can be challenging to accurately identify and correctly diagnose, partly because some intrusive thoughts have very different meanings in non-OCD situations. Common OCD obsessions include intrusive thoughts of stabbing oneself or a loved one, having inappropriate sexual contact with others, or hating God. Parents can understandably be very concerned when their child is having such thoughts, and if a child does not have OCD, these thoughts might be a sign that something else serious is happening with the child, such as being suicidal. When diagnosing OCD, it is very important to understand the child's reaction to the thoughts. With OCD, kids will get very upset by the thoughts because the thoughts seem really bad to them. On the other hand, if the child's thoughts are consistent with how they are feeling in the moment, it is probably not OCD. Let's look at some examples of what is not OCD.

If a child is very sad and having thoughts of cutting or killing themselves with a knife because that feels like the only solution available to them, they are probably experiencing depression, not OCD. Or, if a teenager is very angry and thinking about stabbing the person they are angry with, those thoughts are not OCD but more likely problems with anger control. If a child is starting to become interested in romantic relationships but is unsure how to handle the new feelings of desire and attraction or if a child is questioning the religious beliefs she grew up with, that is probably not OCD but likely a normal developmental phase. In contrast, with OCD, kids might have thoughts of cutting themselves or stabbing their mother when they are happily slicing an apple. Or they may have thoughts that they might be attracted to young children or older relatives, whom they in actuality would never be attracted to. Or they might have thoughts that they don't believe in God when they are otherwise enjoying themselves at Sunday school. In these situations, kids with OCD are so horrified by the thoughts that they use compulsions to get rid of them.

If we are going to be technically correct, OCD is not actually an anxiety disorder. It used to be, but the last time the DSM-5 was updated and published, OCD was moved into its own class of mental health disorders, called the obsessive compulsive and related disorders. One reason for this move was that OCD shows up in a lot of different ways, some of which don't include anxiety as a feature. For some kids, it's more about a situation feeling gross to them—*If I touch that door and pick up germs, I don't think I will get sick, it's just gross to me and I will feel disgusting until I wash the germs off.* Another very common form of OCD is called "just-right" OCD, in which kids feel they have to do something over and over, not to prevent something bad from happening but just so it feels right.

Many anxiety experts continue to combine OCD with anxiety, and we have included OCD in this book for two reasons: There is a lot of overlap between OCD and anxiety disorders, with many kids having OCD and another anxiety disorder, and also exposure therapy is the same recommended treatment for both OCD and anxiety disorders.

Fourteen-year-old Hector had experienced a wide range of OCD symptoms over his childhood, which continued despite various treatments. His symptoms began in second grade with a fear of germs, right after his class was taught the importance of proper hand-washing. Hector became overly concerned about bringing germs home from school, so he started always wearing long-sleeve shirts so he could use his shirtsleeve to open doors. Even doing this, he washed his hands repeatedly until they were red and sore. And when he got home from school, he would avoid touching anything until he had changed into fresh, clean clothes.

Over time his fears of contamination had improved, but he began to have new intrusive thoughts of harming or mistreating others. He feared that if he pointed a part of his body, such as a finger, knee, or elbow, toward someone, that meant he wanted to stab them. He also worried that if he had a thought about hurting someone while doing an action, like picking up a glass or writing a word on a page, then he was likely to act on that thought. In response to these intrusive thoughts, he was constantly paying attention to his body and sitting in uncomfortable positions to avoid pointing any body part at others.

He was also repeating actions, such as standing up and sitting down over and over until he stood up while thinking a safe thought. By the time he started exposure therapy, which finally brought him the help he needed, these thoughts and actions were preventing him from completing his schoolwork or spending time with friends.

### Illness anxiety disorder (hypochondriasis)

Despite its name, illness anxiety disorder is another mental health diagnosis, like OCD, that sits outside anxiety disorders. Illness anxiety disorder is grouped in the somatic symptom and related disorder class in the DSM-5. These mental health disorders include a focus on both medical and physical symptoms. Illness anxiety disorder used to be called hypochondriasis and involves frequent worrying about whether one might have a serious illness. Because illness anxiety disorder is less common in kids than the other anxiety disorders, and since the symptoms (worrying and checking) have a lot of overlap with other anxiety disorders, there is not a chapter in Part 3 of this book devoted to it. Parents of kids with illness anxiety disorder will likely find the chapters on OCD, GAD, and panic disorder most helpful.

Kids who are experiencing illness anxiety disorder often do a lot of checking, which of course is similar to OCD. For example, a teenager might wake up with a headache and begin to worry that she has a brain tumor. So, she might go online and look up brain tumors to see if she has those symptoms. She may then run downstairs and ask her parents if they think she has a brain tumor. The relief she feels when they reassure her that she is healthy is short-lived, and her worrying starts up again soon when the headache returns or she notices another physical symptom.

Sixteen-year-old John's worries focused primarily on his health, particularly concerns that he might have a heart attack. His preoccupation with illness was interfering with his performance at school, since he was so distracted by worries. When his parents took him to see a mental health professional, his mother described John as having always been anxious, cautious, and concerned. However, she traced the increase in his concern about having a heart attack to several years back, when his grandfather went into the hospital for minor heart surgery. Although his grandfather recovered quickly, John began to focus more and more anxiously on his own health. He began checking his pulse several times a day. If he felt his heart begin to beat faster, which is a normal event throughout a teenager's day, he would instantly become nervous and check his pulse again. If this happened at home, he'd ask one of his parents if they thought he was having a heart attack. He researched information about heart disease online, and became nervous if he believed he had a key symptom, such as shortness of breath or chest pain. Due to his increased focus on his body, he became hyper-attuned to small aches, pains, or changes to a degree that even a minor muscle twinge could set off a spiral of worry. When John quit his after-school activities and began spending most of his time at home so his parents could intervene if he had a heart attack, his parents sought help.

## Post-traumatic stress disorder

Post-traumatic stress disorder (PTSD) is a mental health condition in which kids continue to be haunted by nightmares, intense memories, and other symptoms of anxiety long after a traumatic experience has passed. Like OCD, PTSD used to be classified as an anxiety disorder, but is now in its own category of trauma- and stressor-related disorders. Like OCD, we will refer to PTSD in this book because it can also be treated with exposure therapy. However, we won't look too much at PTSD as we don't typically treat it in our anxiety clinic and for that reason discussion of its symptoms will largely fall outside the scope of this book.

Seventeen-year-old Sarah was afraid to get her driver's license. Despite passing the written test, Sarah was unable to complete the behind-the-wheel practice because of an intense fear that she would be in an accident. She and her parents explained that their family had been in a serious car accident about a year and a half earlier. Since beginning driver's education, she had started having nightmares about the accident or causing an accident when driving. For the previous year she had been working hard to distract herself from her worries while riding in the car, but feared that doing so while driving would cause her to lose focus and increase the risk of causing an accident. After learning about PTSD, Sarah started exposure therapy, which helped her see that driving did not automatically segue to an accident, disproving her expectations that an accident was likely.

---

This completes our introduction to the anxiety disorders. We go into each one (except PTSD and illness anxiety) in more detail in Part 3. Our goal for now is for you to begin to match your child's experience and symptoms to one or more of the conditions we've looked at and to feel more confident that we are on the right path. We're now going to build on what we have learned so far by focusing more specifically on understanding your child's experience in a way that sets us up to do exposure therapy.

# 3

# Understanding the Avoidance Cycle

In this chapter we will use what we call the avoidance cycle to help us more precisely understand your child's anxiety in a way that prepares us to treat their symptoms with exposure therapy.

If you're still not sure that the concerns you have about your child match the definition of an anxiety disorder, that's okay. It happens regularly in our clinic that a child's experience just doesn't fit neatly into one of our diagnostic boxes. In those cases, if the family and I think that anxiety treatment is the most reasonable choice, we go ahead and learn about the avoidance cycle to see if it is a good fit for the child's symptoms. If it is, then we keep going. If not, we decide to rule out an anxiety disorder and shift gears to a different mode of treatment.

## THE AVOIDANCE CYCLE

Treating anxiety involves understanding how avoidance is keeping a child or teen stuck in a pattern of fear and worry and then helping them get unstuck. The avoidance cycle is a concept we use in our clinic to help us—the kids, their parents, and our team of mental health professionals—develop a shared understanding of the self-perpetuating loop that is keeping a child feeling anxious.

> Treating anxiety involves understanding how avoidance is keeping a child or teen stuck in a pattern of fear and worry and then helping them get unstuck.

The avoidance cycle has four parts: what sets off a child's fear; what the child expects to happen that makes safe things seem scary; ways of avoiding the source of the fear that prevent the child from learning that their fear and worry are excessive; and the relief from escaping a scary situation that makes it likely the cycle will continue.

First, we'll go through each part of the avoidance cycle, and—because all worries, fears, and OCD symptoms function the same way—we'll use the example of a fear of dogs to illustrate how the avoidance cycle works. Once we understand how avoidance maintains a child's fear of dogs, we can apply the avoidance cycle to your child's fears, worries, obsessions, and compulsions, which work the same way but may not be as straightforward.

Let's go back to Michael from the first chapter and his fear of dogs. Picture him playing happily in his front yard on a sunny summer day. Suddenly, he sees the neighbor across the street open the door and let his dog outside. When Michael sees the dog, he immediately thinks the dog is going to come running across the street and bite him, despite the fact it has never acted in an aggressive way toward him or anyone else. He begins to feel scared and runs back into the house. Once he's inside he feels much better, relieved and also safe because he knows the dog cannot get to him. However, this relief is only temporary because he continues to worry that dogs in general—all dogs—will bite him.

The next time he sees the neighbor's dog, the exact same thing happens; he gets scared and rushes back inside the house. Over time he decides it's too scary to go outside, so he only plays inside, even when it's sunny and his sister wants to go out and run around. This is an example of how an anxiety disorder not only sticks around but can get worse.

With Michael's story in mind, let's go through each part of the avoidance cycle and see how we can use it to understand Michael's experience and how it can apply widely to other kids who don't feel anxious seeing a dog but have other fears and worries or OCD.

## What sets off anxiety (or OCD)

The avoidance cycle begins when something sets off a child's fears or worries. In Michael's case his fear is set off by being around dogs. Although all anxiety disorders and OCD follow the same pattern, each individual child's fears are set off by something different. There are three separate categories of things that can set off anxiety: things around us in the world, thoughts in our head, and feelings in our body. Many kids' anxiety is set off by multiple things from different categories. As we'll see in the second part of this book, understanding what sets off your child's anxiety is really important because that understanding guides what exposure therapy exercises are best suited to treat your child's anxiety. Let's now take a look at each one of those categories.

***Things in the world around us*** Sometimes we are scared of concrete, tangible things around us. This is the case with Michael, whose fear is set off by being near a dog. Other kids might be afraid of bees, mice, or snakes. Children with OCD might have their anxiety set off by objects that might carry germs, like door handles, lunch tables at school, or faucets in public bathrooms. Other kids might have their anxiety set off by being in a certain place or situation, like a park where there might be dogs. Or it could be crowded hallways, riding in an elevator, or staying home alone. Some kids' fears can be set off by certain actions or activities, like starting a conversation, giving a presentation, doing schoolwork, or putting things out of order. Whether anxiety is set off by an object, situation, or activity, all the fears and worries in this category involve an external event kicking off the cycle that leads to a child feeling scared, nervous, or worried. This is the most straightforward category and includes some of the most common sources of anxiety, which are often the easiest to identify. But as you will remember, some forms of anxiety and worry don't seem connected to an external object, situation, or activity. So what sets those avoidance cycles off?

***Thoughts in our head*** Sometimes children feel nervous and worried, even though they are not in a feared situation. Instead, their anxiety is set off by thoughts, such as worries about the future, memories of the past, or OCD obsessions. Returning to the example of Michael, he might start to feel nervous and worried when sitting at home because he starts thinking about visiting his aunt over the weekend and is worried that she might forget to lock the dog in the kennel before they arrive. In this scenario Michael's anxiety is set off by worries about the future. Worries about the future can occur in all anxiety disorders but are one of the most common items that set off anxiety when kids have GAD and might include:

- *I will never get a good job.*
- *I am going to fail this class.*
- *I am going to mess up and we will lose our soccer game.*
- *My friend Zac is going to get mad at me if I miss baseball practice.*

- *Mom is late, I bet she got into an accident.*
- *Someone might break into the house while we're sleeping.*
- *My teacher will get mad if I ask a question.*

Thoughts that set off anxiety can also include memories of things that happened in the past, such as recalling being teased, getting knocked over by a bicycle, seeing a fellow student vomit at school, getting lost in a supermarket, or being pushed over by a bully.

Anxiety-provoking memories are the hallmark of PTSD, but as you can tell from the examples, memories can also set off anxiety for children with other disorders, such as social phobia, specific phobia, or separation anxiety disorder. Michael might get nervous when he remembers a very scary time that a bulldog barked at him at the park. In keeping with our understanding of an anxiety disorder, traumatic events that are recalled in these thoughts need to be in the past and not ongoing, because being anxious about an ongoing upsetting situation is entirely natural and expected and is therefore not a feature of an anxiety disorder but rather a problem in a child's life that needs to be fixed.

The third type of thoughts that set off anxiety are the obsessions or intrusive thoughts that are common with OCD. These are upsetting thoughts that often seem unusual and just pop into a child's mind and won't go away. Examples of this would be a teenager suddenly having a thought like, *I could pick up that knife on the kitchen counter and cut my hand.* A thought like this is crucially not something the child actually wants to do and is frightening to the child because it is very much the opposite of any action they would consider doing.

***Feelings in our body*** For some children, their anxiety occurs even though they are not in a scary situation or thinking scary thoughts.

Rather, their anxiety is set off by feelings they are experiencing within their body. For example, a child may be sitting at home watching a movie when she suddenly notices her heart start to pound or perhaps she gets a sudden stomachache or her chest becomes tight and she finds it hard to breathe. In situations like this the very physical sensations of anxiety or panic set off the child's fears and worries. Children who experience panic disorder or illness anxiety often have their fears and worries set off by symptoms or feelings they experience in their body.

---

Now that we've covered the three categories of things that can set off anxiety and OCD, we should note that many kids' fears can be set off by things from more than one category. A child with separation anxiety might begin to feel frightened by the situation of being alone *or* by the thought that Mom will get into an accident. A child with social anxiety may have her anxiety set off by the activity of talking with people *or* by the memories of awkward social situations. Kids with OCD may feel nervous touching public surfaces *or* when having intrusive thoughts about getting cancer.

It's also important to remember that, in order to meet our definition of an anxiety disorder diagnosis, all the situations, thoughts, or feelings that we identify as setting off the anxiety need to be reasonably safe. "Reasonably" doesn't mean that there is absolutely no chance that the bad thing in question will happen, simply that it is unlikely anything seriously bad will happen, and therefore that most kids would typically be able to handle the situation, thoughts, or feelings. Kids with an anxiety disorder feel more nervous about certain scenarios than we would expect them to feel. So, the feared dog hasn't bitten anyone, the child is not being bullied at school, the child does well on assignments, there have not been recent break-ins, and no one in the family is seriously ill or has recently been in a bad accident. This also applies to OCD thoughts. Cutting oneself is bad, but having a thought about doing that is not dangerous, assuming the child does not want to act on it (which goes back to accurately identifying OCD).

On the other hand, if the situation, thought, or feeling that sets off anxiety is actually dangerous or upsetting to most kids, it is not a sign of anxiety disorder but rather a problem we have to help them fix.

Now that we have a better understanding of what can set off a child's anxiety, we need to understand what makes these safe situations, thoughts, or feelings morph into being so frightening.

## Expectations

Most children are not afraid of dogs. So why do some kids get nervous or terrified around dogs? This is where expectations come in. By expectations we are referring to what a child expects to happen when they are around something, think something, or feel something that sets off their anxiety. These expectations make safe situations feel unsafe. Going back to Michael, he finds dogs scary because he expects them to bite or attack him. Although there are many different expectations that kids can have that make safe situations scary, they generally fall into one of two categories: *Something bad is likely to happen* and *I can't handle this.*

Let's break those two common expectations down.

***Something bad is likely to happen*** When a child expects something bad is going to happen to them or someone they care about, they naturally begin to feel nervous. Michael's belief that the neighbor's dog will bite him is a good example of a child fearing that something bad might happen.

Other expectations along these lines might include:

- *The elevator will get stuck.*
- *I will stumble over my words while giving my presentation in class and people will laugh at me.*
- *My parents won't ever come back from the movies.*
- *If I fail my math test, I will never get a good job.*
- *My heart is pounding, I think I'm having a heart attack.*
- *I've got a bad stomachache, I think I am going to throw up.*
- *These germs will make me get sick and die.*
- *I know my worries about our plane crashing are going to come true, I can feel it.*

If children expect that something bad is likely to happen, then they are going to feel nervous, worried, or scared. While some children have a very specific feared event, other kids have more vague general expectations. For example, some kids with OCD tell us that if they don't walk into their bedroom just right they think their mom will get sick, while others tell us that they have the general sense that something bad is going to happen but can't be more specific. In either case, the child feels nervous because they expect something bad to happen, regardless of how detailed they can be about what that thing is.

***I can't handle this*** Sometimes children of all ages, but especially younger kids, can't point to anything in particular they are afraid will happen and instead just say that the situation, thought, or bodily feeling they're fearful of is simply overwhelming. While some children with OCD fear that germs will make them sick, as mentioned earlier, others believe that germs are just so gross that they won't be able to tolerate the feeling of touching whatever surface carries those germs. In the same way, sometimes children with social anxiety don't actually think that kids will laugh at them or be mean, it's more that talking in a social setting makes them so nervous they believe they just can't do it. Or teens with GAD who tend to worry about lots of different things happening may be convinced that they can't handle the uncertainty of not knowing for sure if things will work out okay.

Children might also expect that a situation will be too upsetting for them to handle alone and that they need their parents to help them get through it. Younger kids with separation anxiety may expect that they will continue to feel scared and upset as long as they are not with their parents, although they may not be able to put their experience into words.

Understanding the expectations your child has that turn safe situations into scary ones is important for treatment planning so we make sure to set up exposures that test and ultimately disprove these expectations.

All of which brings us to a question: Why do Michael and other children with anxiety disorders not learn that their worst-case scenario expectations are unrealistic after their fears repeatedly don't come true? Especially when parents, grandparents, teachers, and even siblings have tried hard to convince them that their fears are unfounded? The answer to this question lies in something we call avoidance.

## Avoidance

The reason that we typically can't talk kids out of an anxiety disorder is that, for all of us, our beliefs and expectations are based on our own lived experiences. If kids are working to avoid all the situations that make them nervous, they never have experiences to disprove their expectations. If every time Michael sees his neighbor's dog he flees inside the house, he never gets to actually find out if

> If kids are working to avoid all the situations that make them nervous, they never have experiences to disprove their expectations.

the dog will bite him or not. If he stayed outside, he would see that the dog sniffs around the lawn and then lies down and takes a big nap in the sun. That would give him the opportunity to realize the dog, at least on this occasion, is harmless. If the same outcome happened the next time, and the next time, and multiple times after that, his expectation that the dog will bite him would be overwhelmed by mounting evidence to the contrary.

Put simply: Avoidance is any action we take to get away from or stop what is bothering us so we feel better or safer. There are three categories of ways that we avoid situations that prevent us from learning that our expectations are actually unlikely to come true: physical avoidance, rituals or overpreparing, and relying on others. We're going to take a closer look at each of these in detail.

***Physical avoidance*** Physical avoidance is the most common form of avoidance and refers to children simply staying as far away as they can from the situation or activity that sets off their anxiety. Sometimes, like Michael going inside when he sees his neighbor's dog, children can entirely avoid the thing they are scared of. In the same way, kids who are very socially anxious might not join extracurricular activities because they will make them nervous to be around other kids. Or kids afraid of elevators get their parents to take the stairs with them.

Sometimes kids can't avoid the whole situation, and so they just avoid as much as possible. Those socially anxious kids who avoid joining extracurricular activities might also like to avoid going to school, but their parents won't allow it. So, when they are at school they avoid as much social interaction as they can by keeping their eyes down, leaving the classroom as fast as possible so no one has the chance to talk to them, only asking questions of a classmate they know well, and when they are asked a question, answering quickly and quietly and moving on before the person can ask something else. So even though they don't avoid going to school, they get through the day by avoiding as much of the feared social interactions as they can.

When a kid's anxiety is set off by thoughts in their head, like worries about the future, they might mentally avoid by distracting themselves. A child who is very worried that their parents are late getting home because they were in a car accident might try to read or play video games to distract them from these worry thoughts.

***Rituals and overpreparing*** Another way children avoid anxiety-provoking situations when actual physical avoidance is not possible is by doing rituals or overpreparing. Rituals are a common form of avoidance in OCD. When kids do rituals, they are either trying to fix things to avoid something bad happening or to avoid feeling overwhelmed. For example, children who are afraid of germs might avoid touching public surfaces but when they do have to use a door handle, they do rituals like washing their hands excessively to avoid any chance of getting sick. Or if kids are afraid they've forgotten to pack their homework, they might repeatedly check their backpack to avoid the distress of not knowing for sure if they forgot their homework. A girl with OCD who fears that walking through a doorway while thinking about her grandfather having a stroke will actually cause him to have a stroke may try to avoid this feared outcome by walking back and forth through the doorway until she can do so with a safe alternative thought, like *Grandpa is fine.* This ritual allows her to avoid her perception that she is the cause of her grandfather's stroke and avoid feeling the distress from uncertainty.

Another way children take action to avoid anxious distress or potential problems is overpreparing. If a child feels anxious about ordering food at a restaurant because he is afraid he may mispronounce the dish he wants and the waitress will laugh at him, then before ordering he might rehearse how to pronounce the pasta dish he wants repeatedly in his head to avoid any chance of making a mistake.

Overpreparing is a common form of avoidance for kids with GAD who worry about their academic performance. Some kids, like Kara, despite being straight-A students, worry about their grades. They constantly worry that they will get a bad grade on the next assignment or fail an upcoming test. To avoid the possibility of doing poorly they overprepare by rechecking their work multiple times, writing essay answers that are twice as long as they need to be, studying extra hours long after demonstrating that they clearly know the material for the test, or doing extra credit when they already have a 100% in the class. Frequently, this overpreparation comes at the expense of sleep, downtime, family activities, and friendships.

***Relying on others*** A third way that children avoid situations, thoughts, or feelings that cause them distress is by relying on other people, which typically means leaning on their parents. This may take the form of kids asking a parent repeatedly for reassurance that something bad won't happen, in order to avoid handling the worries on their own. John, the 16-year-old teenager with health anxiety, might ask his mom over and over and over again if she thinks the stomachaches he is experiencing mean he has an ulcer. Seeking his mother's reassurance that he is fine allows John to briefly avoid the distress of worrying that he does have an ulcer.

Alex, the 8-year-old who worries about his parents' safety, might frequently call or text his dad to check that his parents are okay after they go out on a date night, because his Dad's response that yes they are fine and enjoying dinner helps Alex avoid the distress of worrying that they have been injured in an accident. Or he might insist on having a parent lie beside him in bed until he falls asleep to avoid handling nervousness alone. Or he may cling to his parents, cry, get angry, or have a tantrum when being dropped off at school or left with a babysitter, to prevent or delay that separation and fear that comes with being away from his parents.

For children with social anxiety, relying on others might include having their parents, siblings, or friends order food, make phone calls, ask directions, talk to a teacher, or answer questions for them. This allows the child to avoid the distress of speaking in social situations and heads off the possibility of saying something embarrassing.

Children with contamination fears may demand that their parents do extra laundry unnecessarily or wash their hands frequently when preparing meals.

---

As we mentioned at the beginning of this section, for all of us, our beliefs and expectations are based on our own experience. Unfortunately, all of these forms of avoidance—physical, rituals and overpreparation, relying on others—prevent kids having their own experiences to learn that their fears are unlikely to happen and that they can handle feeling anxious.

Recognizing what kids are doing to avoid their fears is crucial to making a successful exposure treatment plan. Specifically, when your child does exposures, they need to stop avoiding and doing rituals because that avoidance will prevent them from learning the situation is not as dangerous as they expected. If your child continues avoidance during exposures, they will believe that the activity turned out okay only because they avoided the worst part, or fixed it by ritualizing, or had your help to get them through.

Now you may be wondering, if avoidance keeps the problem going, why do kids keep avoiding it? Why does Michael keep running inside when he sees the neighbor's dog, even though this means he is going to continue to feel nervous or worried and miss out on fun things like playing outside? The answer to this question is something called reinforcement.

## Relief is reinforcing

*Reinforcement* is a more complicated term for a reward, something that we enjoy, something that makes us feel good. A basic principle of learning and behavior change is that if something good happens after we do something, we will probably do that same thing again.

Most parents are familiar with this idea and use rewards, like a new toy or video game time, to encourage kids to do tasks like chores or homework. It turns out that removing something unpleasant is also rewarding or, if we want to be fancy, reinforcing. Your baby crying nonstop in public is an unpleasant and upsetting experience. If your baby stops crying when you pick him up and feed him, you have just been rewarded by the removal of something distressing. An end to the unpleasant crying makes you feel relieved and encourages you to feed your baby quickly the next time he cries.

We have a similar experience in the avoidance cycle. Nobody likes to feel scared and nervous. Anything we do that makes us feel better, like getting away from a scary situation, is automatically reinforced, so we do it more. The relief Michael feels when he runs inside to escape the neighbor's dog is rewarding, because once inside he feels safe—he's escaped the threat of the German shepherd's jaws—so he keeps running inside whenever he sees the dog. Running away has proven to be a quick way to feel better immediately.

However, the rewarding nature of relief not only keeps kids stuck in the avoidance cycle; it can also make their problems with fear and worry get worse over time. Michael might start out avoiding his neighbor's dog but because running inside the house works so well to feel better, he might start to also run away when he sees any dog. Eventually, this might lead him to avoid going to places where a dog might be encountered—neighborhood streets, the local park, or new friends' houses. Relief starts to look like a world with no dogs.

Similarly, the relief a child with OCD feels after washing germs from a doorknob off her hands encourages her to wash her hands more frequently and after touching an increasing number of items beyond doorknobs and handles. Or in the case of separation anxiety, the child who keeps messaging his mom and dad on their date night and getting a response that tells him they are okay will keep doing it and start messaging, perhaps from the restrooms at school, to check if they are okay at work too.

Recognizing the immediate reinforcing power of relief from avoiding anxiety-provoking situations is important for understanding what motivates a child to keep avoiding in the face of mounting problems associated with an anxiety disorder. For parents, this understanding can turn a frustrating and at times incomprehensible behavior pattern into an understandable and predictable response to the desire we all have for immediate relief from distress.

## THE CYCLE CONTINUES

As we've now seen, children with anxiety disorders who consistently avoid the situations, thoughts, and feelings that make them nervous never have enough experiences to rewrite their expectations. In the absence of opportunities to learn something new, they continue to expect either that bad things will happen or that they cannot handle the situations they fear. And so naturally, the next time they encounter the situation, thoughts, or feelings that set off their anxiety before, the same old avoidance kicks into action again and the same old expectations remain untested. Although Michael feels better once he has gotten away from his neighbor's dog, he still believes that dogs are dangerous and likely to bite him and what's more, he's terrified thinking about where he might run into a dog. The next time he sees his neighbor's dog, or any other dog, the avoidance cycle repeats itself, as if on a loop. Children with anxiety disorders find themselves trapped in this never-ending cycle of getting anxious, avoiding, feeling temporarily relieved, worrying about the next time, and then having it repeat again. This is the cycle we need to break if we are going to help our anxious children feel better.

Children with anxiety disorders find themselves trapped in this never-ending cycle of getting anxious, avoiding, feeling temporarily relieved, worrying about the next time, and then having it repeat again. This is the cycle we need to break if we are going to help our anxious children feel better.

## HOW DID IT START?

You might have noticed that the anxiety cycle doesn't address what started a child's fears and worries in the first place. Parents understandably come to our clinic wanting to know why their child is suffering from fear and worry and where their child's problems with anxiety come from. The answer is that like most characteristics, anxiety disorders are partly genetic or inherited and partly based on our own experiences. This is often called nature (genetics and hereditary factors) and nurture (environmental and circumstantial factors).

As a rule of thumb, when it comes to nature, many anxious children have anxious parents. Most of our characteristics are inherited: hair color, eye color, height. Many of our basic traits have a genetic component—even personality. And anxiety disorders are no different: anxious parents

Anxiety disorders are partly genetic or inherited and partly based on our own experiences.

tend to have anxious kids. Genes do not give the full answer though. Plenty of anxious parents raise children who do not have anxiety disorders. And plenty of anxious kids have non-anxious parents. But having a parent with an anxiety disorder will increase the odds of a child having an anxiety disorder too.

On the nurture aspect, a child's experience is also important in understanding how an anxiety disorder developed. The avoidance cycle that we just learned about explains how fears and worries can grow and become more problematic over time. It is seldom clear what initially started the avoidance cycle in motion. Some kids and parents can point to a specific event, such as bullying or teasing at school leading to social anxiety disorder, seeing a classmate throw up leading to a specific phobia of vomiting, or learning about the importance of hand-washing in health class leading to contamination OCD. And other times a stressful or traumatic event leads to anxiety.

However, it is more common for there not to be any clear event or reason behind the onset of anxiety. Rather, parents often tell us that their child has always been nervous and it just got worse over time. In general, we don't know why a child begins to have an anxiety disorder. For any given child we can't say what combination of genetics and previous experiences are the cause. And in some ways it doesn't particularly matter, since there is nothing any of us can do to go back and change a child's genetics or previous experiences.

What matters is what is happening now. Working together, we can change the ongoing pattern of behavior that is maintaining the anxiety disorder. This is where the avoidance cycle comes in. It is how we understand the current circumstances that are keeping a child stuck in an anxiety disorder or OCD. Once we understand what maintains the cycle, we can break it and help kids feel braver and calmer. We can successfully do that whether or not a child has inherited an anxious personality from their parents or experienced a scary event that started the whole thing off.

---

The goal of this chapter was to use the avoidance cycle to understand how your child's expectations make safe situations scary, how avoidance prevents those fears from going away, and how reinforcement makes it likely to happen again. Understanding how your child's experience fits in the avoidance cycle helps us to tailor treatment to reduce their anxiety by breaking the cycle with exposure therapy. Before we start talking about anxiety treatment though, we need to make sure we haven't overlooked other emotions and behaviors that might be important. To that end, we need to be certain that there is nothing else that better explains your child's symptoms or would get in the way of treating their anxiety.

# 4

# What Else Could It Be?

Children are complex and can't be defined by just one trait, including anxiety. Even if by this point you are confident that your child is experiencing an anxiety disorder, there might be other things going on as well. Sometimes depression or anger outbursts need to be addressed first, before we can successfully treat anxiety or OCD.

On the other hand, you might still be unsure whether the concerns you have about your child are best described by an anxiety disorder. If so, it can be helpful to see if another category of mental health problems better describes your child's difficulties. Should that be the case, then we can shift the plan accordingly. For these reasons, before we start talking about treatment with exposure therapy, we are going to review other common mental health problems that might be confused for or complicate anxiety disorders and OCD.

It is probably helpful to keep in mind that identifying the most accurate diagnosis when a child has a variety of emotional and behavioral symptoms is challenging, even for medical and mental health professionals. So, don't feel as if you need to become an expert on all the various conditions we explore. Rather, if one of these categories seems like it could be a good fit for your child's symptoms, we should probably explore some other treatment options before or while we work on anxiety.

## OTHER MENTAL HEALTH CONDITIONS

Children can experience more than one mental health condition at a time. Kids with anxiety may have other behavioral or emotional difficulties that can interfere with or prevent us from working on their anxiety disorder. We call these comorbid conditions.

> Kids with anxiety may have other behavioral or emotional difficulties that can interfere with or prevent us from working on their anxiety disorder.

When children are experiencing more than one mental health problem, which is very common, we often have to decide which problem we are going to treat first. In general, mental health professionals and families begin by working on the problem that is most concerning to the family or causing the biggest problems in the child's daily life.

Less often, we need to work on a different problem first—not the most pressing and obvious—even though it is not the family's biggest concern, because its symptoms will prevent us from working on the primary condition.

Let's take a look at some common behavioral and emotional problems that could be misidentified as an anxiety disorder or disrupt successful exposure therapy for an anxiety disorder.

### Adjustment to stress

Kids can feel anxious, as well as sad and angry, when they are having difficulty adjusting to a big change in their life or a stressful life event. There are many different events that can lead to stress in childhood, including family conflict, parental separation, contracting a serious illness, being in an accident, the death of a loved one, a family member contracting a prolonged illness, bullying, discrimination, changing schools, and academic problems.

When a child experiences such an event, we expect them to have a reaction, and that reaction often includes fear and worry. However, that fear and worry is understandable. If a child worries about what life will be like after their parents' divorce or after a grandparent passes away from illness, then the appropriate treatment is to strengthen support through that difficult transition. If a child is nervous about school because they are being bullied or failing their classes, then the appropriate treatment is to help find a solution to fix those problems.

Kids feeling nervous and worried during a stressful time is different from having an anxiety disorder. When kids have an anxiety disorder, they are more nervous, worried, or scared about something than we would expect. This is because they are expecting something bad to happen that turns safe situations into scary ones despite the fact that nothing unusually stressful or upsetting is currently happening in the child's life to cause their anxiety. In contrast, when kids are adjusting to stress, they will have recently experienced something upsetting.

> It is important to clearly identify the difference between excessive fear and worry that we will need to treat with exposure therapy and expected fear and worry in response to a stressful situation that needs to be addressed with support and problem-solving.

Children who have a stressful life, perhaps with family financial problems or parents fighting regularly at home, can also have an anxiety disorder. Sometimes what starts out as a natural anxiety response to a stressful situation, financial problems, or family conflict morphs into excessive fear and worry even though the problems or fighting get resolved. In these cases, anxiety specific to a stressful period in life goes on to calcify into an anxiety disorder long after the stress has passed.

It is important to clearly identify the difference between excessive fear and worry that we will need to treat with exposure therapy and expected fear and worry in response to a stressful situation that needs to be addressed with support and problem-solving.

## Depression

It's not uncommon for kids who experience anxiety disorders to also experience depression. Sometimes it's because the anxiety disorder is the primary problem, has been around longer, and has caused or led over time to depression. Let's take 16-year-old Maria, who has social anxiety. Her anxiety interferes with her ability to participate in activities and make new friends and has made school stressful. Over time, she becomes sad and down because she's missing out on fun activities that she sees other kids at school enjoying. She feels isolated, which leads to depression. Of course, it's also possible that depression can be present before anxiety or that they develop independently.

One treatment for depression is behavioral activation, which simply means helping children to increase the number of activities in their lives that improve their mood and help them feel happier. Those activities can include physical exercise, enjoyable social activities, and activities that lead to a sense of success, like a hobby, job, or schoolwork.

There can be a significant overlap in how we treat anxiety and depression. For social anxiety, we do exposure therapy around talking to people—things like starting conversations, making plans, speaking up in class, ordering in restaurants. Successfully completing these exposures can lead to a sense of accomplishment, and some of these exposures involve fun social activities. For these reasons, we often don't have to choose between treating anxiety or depression, because treatment for one often helps the other at the same time.

Due to that overlap, we recommend treating an anxiety disorder with exposure therapy unless symptoms of depression are severe enough to interfere with treatment. When children are severely depressed, they often feel badly about themselves, low in energy, and hopeless: symptoms that can make it difficult to participate in exposure therapy by robbing kids of their motivation and making it hard for them to have faith that doing these exercises will help. Most importantly, if children are having suicidal thoughts, we need to make sure they are safe by having a safety plan in place detailing how they will be supervised and what they will do if they feel like hurting themselves. In these cases, we then need to help improve their mood before we start exposure therapy for their fear and worries.

## Anger and defiance

It's fairly common for children to get angry and argumentative when asked to do something that makes them nervous. This is part of the fight or flight response that we learned about earlier. This is so common that our standard treatment for anxiety disorders includes strategies to address these problems, which we call the motivation plan.

Sometimes though, outbursts of anger and lack of cooperation become a bigger obstacle. This can happen when anxiety-related outbursts are very intense and happen frequently or when defiance around feared situations starts to spread to defiance around other unpleasant but not scary situations, like chores.

Some children have a general tendency to be argumentative and defiant, and if there has been a long-standing pattern of frequent, excessive, and problematic arguing, refusing to do what's asked of them, angry outbursts, blaming others for their mistakes, and irritability, then this may be oppositional defiant disorder (ODD). Since anger outbursts and resistant behaviors commonly occur in childhood, we only diagnose this disorder if symptoms are excessive and problematic.

Anger and defiance, whether confined to anxiety situations or as part of ODD, make it more difficult to treat an anxiety disorder. If children generally argue and refuse to do things that are unpleasant but not particularly challenging, like turning off video games, cleaning up their room, or getting ready for school, it is likely that they will be argumentative and resistant to doing exposure therapy, which they know will be unpleasant and challenging. As such, when children are being argumentative and defiant, we focus on establishing cooperation first, before we try to address anxiety through exposure therapy.

The standard treatment, and the one we use in our clinic, to increase cooperation and address ODD specifically is called behavior management. This involves working with parents to use firm and reasonable expectations to make it clear what kids need to do to be successful; positive attention and tangible rewards to encourage kids to engage in positive, good behaviors; and ignoring and consequences to discourage misbehavior.

Many parents are familiar with basic behavior management, such as sticker charts and time-outs. When anger and defiance become more problematic, parents have to become expert at using behavior management strategies more consistently and precisely than parents typically do.

At our clinic we work with parents to help them understand and get the most out of these strategies, and we support them as they deploy the strategies over time. Once cooperation has improved, then parents can extend their system of clear expectations, rewards, and consequences to ensure cooperation with exposure therapy.

One nice benefit of beginning with behavior management is that these strategies can be very effective for improving a wide variety of concerns parents have about their children. If you are still not sure whether your child's experience is best described by an anxiety disorder, one option is to start with behavior management.

Let's say your child complains about not feeling well in the morning, acts anxious, and resists getting ready for school. While it seems like they might be worried and nervous about school, based on what you've read in this book so far, their symptoms may not really fit with what we have learned about anxiety disorders. If this is you and your child right now, you can start off by giving your child specific goals to act calmly and cooperatively in the morning and use rewards and consequences to motivate their efforts. You may find this intervention is all you need. If not, then going through this process may give you a better understanding of your child's fears and worries that would be best addressed through exposure therapy.

## ADHD

Many parents are aware of attention deficit/hyperactivity disorder (ADHD). ADHD involves two sets of symptoms: inattention and hyperactivity/impulsivity. Inattention includes: making careless mistakes, being distractible, leaving activities unfinished, having difficulty remaining focused, being disorganized, and losing things. Hyperactivity/impulsivity includes: being fidgety and squirmy, having a constant restless energy and activity as if driven by a motor, displaying difficulty waiting one's turn, and showing a tendency toward interrupting others. When children have ADHD, these symptoms interfere with schoolwork, chores, and completing daily activities.

Just as kids with ADHD have difficulties concentrating and focusing on schoolwork, they may face the same challenges with exposure therapy and find themselves getting fidgety, restless, and distracted. When ADHD symptoms interfere with completing exposure therapy for anxiety disorders, they should, ideally, be treated first.

Sometimes ADHD symptoms can lead to situational stress that looks a lot like an anxiety disorder. Children with ADHD may be frequently reprimanded at school for being impulsive and not sitting still, which may lead them to worry about getting in trouble at school. Or they may be having difficulties with friendships because their impulsivity or high activity level causes conflict with peers. Or they may feel overwhelmed by schoolwork because getting easily distracted makes homework take an extra-long time. They may be worried about tests, because they have trouble focusing in class and when studying, which leaves them unprepared for tests. In this case, the goal is not to try and reduce the child's anxiety about the real problems they are having at school but to help get those problems under control through successfully treating their ADHD. Sometimes successfully treating ADHD can resolve symptoms that appeared at first to be an anxiety disorder.

To make matters more complicated, symptoms of anxiety can also sometimes look like ADHD. When children are worried and nervous in school they might find it difficult to focus, make decisions, and complete schoolwork on time. In these cases, we should treat the anxiety first and see if the problems with attention improve with the reduced worry.

One way to sort out whether anxiety or ADHD is the root cause of problems with attention is to look at areas where the symptoms don't overlap. If worry is causing a child to lose focus, we would expect to see that child getting very nervous and worried in a variety of situations, including situations that are not related to focusing on schoolwork. Likewise, if lack of focus is causing worry, we would expect the child to be easily distracted even at times that don't cause worry, such as playing board games at home.

Of course, there are times when, despite our best efforts, it is still not clear whether a child has problems with anxiety or ADHD or both. When we don't feel confident whether anxiety or ADHD is the root cause, one option is to begin anxiety treatment. The process of completing the avoidance cycle, then planning and doing exposure therapy, can clarify whether an anxiety disorder is the principal cause of what the child is experiencing.

Another option is to start with behavior management as we described above under anger and defiance and see if this improves the concerning behaviors through clear expectations, rewards, and consequences. If a behavioral therapy approach is successful, then additional treatment may not be needed. However, if problems with attention, hyperactivity, or impulsivity interfere with the success of exposure therapy or behavior management, this information can be useful in diagnosing ADHD. Treatment of ADHD involves a thorough evaluation to make sure the diagnosis is accurate and then working with a psychiatrist or other medical doctor for medication management. Behavior management can also be helpful to provide more structure for kids with ADHD.

## Difficulties managing emotions and self-harm

Successfully completing treatment for anxiety requires managing distress during exposure therapy until the fear or worry decreases. It also requires working cooperatively with other people, whether it is the therapist, parents, other kids, or teachers during exposures.

When children find it hard to manage emotions or handle relationships in general, these challenges can interfere with exposure therapy. In addition, problematic emotional reactions and interpersonal stress can lead to anxiety, worry, and distress.

Kids with anxiety disorders may certainly become very upset in situations that provoke their fears and worries, and their reactions can be intense. However, some children have intense reactions around many different types of situations, involving the full range of emotions from sadness to frustration and anger.

> When children find it hard to manage emotions or handle relationships in general, these challenges can interfere with exposure therapy. In addition, problematic emotional reactions and interpersonal stress can lead to anxiety, worry, and distress.

Kids with difficulties managing emotions may become very angry when things don't go their way. They and their families often describe their emotions as unpredictable, unstable, and variable. The child is very happy and then suddenly inconsolably upset. Their relationships with others can be rocky, as they frequently get mad at their friends or, in the snap of a finger, feel like everybody hates them. When children have difficulties managing relationships and intense emotions, they may intentionally hurt themselves, such as by cutting their arms or legs; slapping, pinching, or punching themselves; or burning their arms or legs with a match or lighter, as a way to numb and override overwhelming feelings. They may also have suicidal thoughts or feel like they would rather be dead when they are upset.

Fear and worry may certainly be a problem for these children. But sometimes that fear and worry is a reaction to a pattern of emotional outbursts that have damaged relationships. Other times, they may have an anxiety disorder, but the emotional ups and downs and intense reactions they routinely experience are likely to interfere with exposure therapy because when they get distressed, they lash out at others or themselves. For kids whose experience fits this description, we need to give them skills to help them manage their distress and better navigate relationships in times of stress before we can treat their fears and worries with exposure therapy.

## Autism spectrum disorder

Autism spectrum disorder (ASD) is a mental health diagnosis, increasingly referred to as a neurodevelopmental disorder, that involves three primary areas of difficulties. First, kids with ASD find social interactions challenging and confusing because it's hard for them to understand or pick up on subtle forms of communication such as facial expressions or changes in tone of voice. Second, children diagnosed with ASD tend toward rigidity, black-and-white thinking, and inflexibly adhering to certain routines. Children may become very upset if their routine changes, even one that doesn't necessarily make sense, such as always eating a certain cereal from a specific bowl while sitting in a specific chair. Children with ASD may also have highly narrow, special interests, such as an exhaustive passion for locomotives, whales, or space travel, and will talk about these interests nonstop without interruption, even if others are not interested or become visibly irritated. Third, children with ASD tend also to have sensory sensitivities such as not tolerating tags in shirts, the seams in socks, or the feel of blue jeans. Kids might also overreact to sounds or smells or be unreactive or insensitive to pain. Historically, an autism diagnosis was limited to children with high levels of impairment who were often unable to function independently, but since the DSM-5, autism has been increasingly viewed as a cluster of traits occurring on a spectrum that includes some children who are successful academically, with their most observable difficulty being navigating social and emotional relationships.

Children with ASD may experience high levels of anxiety. However, it is important to separate fears and worries that constitute an anxiety disorder from fears and worries that result from symptoms of ASD. If kids with ASD get nervous about social situations because they don't have the conversation skills to be successful, this is likely related to ASD, and we should help them learn how to start and hold conversations so they can be more successful in social situations. On the other hand, if a child with ASD is very nervous about giving a presentation despite typically doing well, then we would approach this as an anxiety disorder and treat their fear with exposure therapy.

Some kids with ASD also engage in repetitive behaviors and/or follow rigid routines that can appear similar to OCD rituals. However, when these actions are reflective of ASD symptoms, they typically revolve around something the child prefers to do, such as repeatedly talking about a favorite topic, wanting sameness in routines, or what is often referred to as stimming (a term deriving from self-stimulating), which is when autistic children might flap their hands, clap, or rock backward and forward. In contrast, as we learned earlier, children with OCD do not want to engage in their repetitive routine behaviors and rituals at all. Instead, they feel compelled to do so to relieve distress.

Kids with ASD who also have anxiety disorders can very much benefit from exposure therapy. However, completing exposures means tolerating distress and learning in the moment that a fear is not going to come true. If a child with ASD tends to be emotionally reactive and think rigidly, the pace of treatment may need to be slowed down and the child given additional support to help manage their emotions and think flexibly.

## Eating and weight concerns

When children experience anxiety at the same time as changes in eating habits and appetite, it may be necessary to address their basic health before beginning exposure therapy for an anxiety disorder.

In general, if a child or teenager is not eating enough to maintain their typical weight, their eating habits and weight need to be restored before they are likely to be successful with exposure therapy. This can be true even when anxiety has led to weight loss, like when children have difficulty eating due to a specific phobia of throwing up or OCD concerns about food becoming contaminated.

If anxiety has merely made it harder to eat, because the child's stomach is in knots, yet their weight has not changed very much, we would begin exposure therapy to address the anxiety that is interfering with eating.

However, if the child has lost substantial weight, even as a result of anxiety, the child might not be ready for exposure therapy. In this context, by "underweight" we are referring to the child's weight relative to what is normal for that child. You can ask your general physician if you need expert guidance. Generally speaking, children can be healthy at average, lower, or higher weight percentiles compared to their peers. However, when a child's weight is generally at the 70th percentile and then it drops to the 50th, or from the 50th to the 30th, or from the 30th to the 10th, that may be a cause for concern and requires medical consultation.

There are a couple of reasons why it is important to address eating and weight before anxiety. When children are not eating enough to sustain their typical body weight, it can affect the way they feel. Kids may feel anxious or distressed or just physically uncomfortable. These feelings may also be accompanied by becoming more emotionally reactive and getting very upset or tearful or angry or sad or anxious more quickly and intensely than they have in the past. Although their anxious distress and tearfulness may look similar to an anxiety disorder, it might be more of a result from reduced eating and weight change. Rather than needing exposure, these kids need to return to their previous eating habits; as their weight restores, mood-related symptoms will often resolve.

Even when children clearly have an anxiety disorder, such as a fear of food being contaminated, accompanied by substantial weight loss, exposure therapy is often not successful without a weight restoration program first. When kids are substantially below weight, in addition to being more easily upset and having difficulty managing emotions they can become more rigid and have difficulty thinking flexibly. As we discussed above, successful exposure therapy involves managing distress and shifting one's expectations as the child comes to see that when they face their fears, what they were afraid of doesn't actually occur. This can be difficult to do when low weight has a child running on empty. In such cases, restoring weight first sets kids up to be successful with exposure therapy.

## Physical and medical symptoms

When children are anxious, they may have stomachaches, headaches, muscle tightness, or pain. Younger kids in particular may express anxiety by saying they don't feel well and have a stomachache. However, other times kids experience chronic and persistent pain, such as headaches, stomachaches, and joint pain as well as other physical symptoms such as dizziness, nausea, and fatigue. Not only are these physical symptoms distressing, they can also significantly interfere with a child's ability to go to school, socialize, or even get up in the morning to do daily activities.

There are various ways that chronic pain and physical symptoms, like dizziness or fatigue, can interact with anxiety. When children are experiencing chronic pain or fatigue, they may begin to be nervous about going somewhere because they don't want to have a headache while they're there. They might also worry about their future and whether their recurring pain will resolve over time and if not, whether they will be able to function when they grow up. Other children may have had problems with anxiety before they developed the pain, and not only are those fears and worries still around but they add another layer of distress surrounding the physical pain that makes it even more difficult to function.

The treatment for chronic pain and other physical symptoms begins with a thorough medical evaluation to address any underlying health problems. When medical treatments can't fully resolve chronic pain and fatigue, treatment may then include what are called biobehavioral pain management strategies, such as relaxation, mindfulness, and therapy to help kids limit how often pain interferes with functioning.

When children have both anxiety and chronic physical symptoms, often the decision regarding which to treat first comes down to which is interfering most with the child's everyday life. Treatment for anxiety is active and requires being able to participate in exposure therapy at a clinic, at home, and in real-world settings, like school and with peers. If a child's headaches, fatigue, or other physical symptoms are going to interfere with or prevent them from doing exposure therapy, those symptoms need to be addressed first. Similarly, if a child's fears and worries focus mostly on the possibility of having pain, especially at times when it would be difficult to manage that pain, such as at school, these worries often come true because the child actually does experience pain. In this instance, the pain needs to be addressed first.

## Substance use

Substance use is another mental health condition that typically needs to be addressed before working on an anxiety disorder. If kids are using alcohol, marijuana, or illegal drugs or misusing prescription medication, this can result in agitation, mood fluctuation, depression, paranoia, panic attacks, and anxiety. While some of these symptoms can be described as similar to those of an anxiety disorder, it is difficult to separate which symptoms are a side effect of the substance use and which are a sign of an anxiety disorder. Moreover, use of alcohol and drugs can also cause social and academic difficulties that result in anxiety and distress.

### Severe mental illness onset

Some children may unfortunately have early signs of a severe and persistent mental illness that may include symptoms of feeling anxious or worried. Other symptoms that would raise concerns for the onset of a severe mental health condition include delusional beliefs; becoming very disorganized; losing interest in taking care of oneself, such as not showering or changing clothes; episodes of mania; and other erratic, unusual behavior. In this case, it is important to take your child for a thorough psychiatric evaluation, especially if there is a family history of severe mental illness.

---

The previous chapters focused on different ways to understand what an anxiety disorder *is,* while this chapter has focused on what *is not* an anxiety disorder. Understanding what is not an anxiety disorder helps us when we are on the fence about whether a child's experience is best described as an anxiety disorder or OCD. Sometimes, knowing what else to call the symptoms that a child is experiencing makes it easier to decide that it is not an anxiety disorder or OCD.

It also helps us have a comprehensive understanding of a child's experience. Kids with anxiety disorders often have other emotional and behavioral symptoms. A full view of other common mental health conditions and how they might affect anxiety disorder treatment helps us decide what to focus on first. Ideally, this chapter has helped you decide whether your child is experiencing other symptoms that need to be addressed instead of or before working on their anxiety.

## PART 1 CONCLUSION

At this point I hope you feel confident in your analysis of whether your child is more afraid and nervous than we would expect of certain things, places, thoughts, or bodily feelings; whether their fears and worries are similar to one or more of the anxiety disorders we have looked at; whether their experience fits within the avoidance cycle that explains how problematic anxiety is maintained; and whether another mental health condition better describes your child's experience or will interfere with anxiety treatment.

This is a good time to sit down with your child to talk about anxiety and see if your child feels that anxiety accurately describes their experience. It's okay if you and your child see things differently and don't agree. Kids and parents have different perspectives and may disagree about whether a child is experiencing an anxiety disorder and how serious it is. In my experience, both perspectives are important and need to be listened to. Sometimes, kids are right and what parents think is anxiety is really more the kids' preferences, and it might be the parents' anxiety that is driving their concern. Sometimes, parents are right, and kids are denying that their anxiety is a problem because they are so nervous they don't even want to talk about it. And sometimes the truth is somewhere in between.

I don't expect you at this stage in the book to have arrived at a specific diagnosis for the concerns you have about your child. After all, an actual mental health diagnosis requires an evaluation by a medical or mental health professional. But if you feel pretty confident that the concept of an anxiety disorder seems to be the most likely way to describe and understand your child's experience, then let's proceed to Part 2 of this book, where we will learn what exposure therapy is and how to treat your child's anxiety or OCD with it.

If, on the other hand, you're still not feeling confident that problems with anxiety best describe the concerns you have about your child, then I recommend you seek professional help at this point. Most families begin the mental health journey by meeting with their child's pediatrician or family doctor. If your child is already meeting with a therapist or counselor, you can also talk with them to make sure they agree with how you now understand your child's symptoms.

# PART 2

## An Introduction to Exposure Therapy

In the first part of this book, we learned about anxiety disorders and OCD, how to recognize each of them, and whether one or more disorders describes your child's experience. We're now going to learn how we treat anxiety disorders and OCD by helping kids face their fears using exposure therapy. First, we're going to look at the history and evidence behind exposure therapy, then describe what exposures entail, highlight the best track for your success, and move on to laying out a step-by-step plan for setting up, doing, and ending an exposure. We'll also spotlight how you as a parent, guardian, or caregiver are an essential part of the process. To finish up, we'll lay out a suggested timeline for what exposure therapy might look like from start to finish.

My goal by that point is for you to feel confident that you understand what exposure therapy is and why it is the most appropriate treatment for your child's fears and worries. In Part 3 we'll start building specific treatment plans for the anxiety symptoms your child experiences.

It is important to say that reading this book won't make you an expert on exposure therapy, but it can help you feel more confident to coach your child through exposure therapy at home or to look for a therapist with the right expertise.

# 5

# The Origins of Exposure Therapy

Treating anxiety disorders with exposure therapy involves the child facing their fears and learning through lived experience that what they are afraid of is unlikely to happen and that they can in fact handle feeling anxious. The rationale for using exposure therapy arises from how we understand anxiety disorders and how your child's fears fit into the avoidance cycle.

To recap, with an anxiety disorder kids are more nervous, worried, or afraid of a situation than we would expect them to be because they expect something bad will happen that they cannot handle. By avoiding the situation or doing rituals, they never get the chance to learn that the situation they fear isn't as bad as they thought it would be and that they can in fact manage it. Avoidance provides relief in the moment but keeps kids trapped in a cycle of fear and avoidance. Exposure therapy breaks this cycle.

To illustrate what we mean, let's catch up again with 10-year-old Michael and his fear of dogs. Michael is playing in the front yard when suddenly his neighbor's dog barrels out the front door.

As before, Michael immediately thinks the dog is going to bite him and becomes afraid. But this is where things change. Rather than running inside like he used to do, this time Michael decides to face his fear. He stays outside in his yard and watches as the dog runs across the neighbor's lawn to inspect a tree, turns around, and starts barking at him. After about ten seconds of barking, the dog quiets down, stretches out, and lies down on the grass. All this time Michael stands still, his heart pounding. Slowly the pounding in his chest settles and his anxiety eases. He realizes the dog is not going to bite him and isn't even all that interested in him. By remaining in the yard and facing his fears, Michael took an initial step toward breaking the cycle of avoidance that had, until now, prevented him from enjoying playing outside like other kids. This scenario illustrates a fundamental principle of exposure—Michael took action despite his anxiety. He stayed outside and changed his usual pattern of behavior first, and only after that began to feel better.

Doing something that makes your child feel scared is essential for exposure therapy to work. It would be infinitely easier if kids could stop worrying and feeling scared first and then face their fears. But unfortunately, it doesn't work that way, because we can't control our thoughts and feelings. We can, with dedicated effort, control our actions. And if we take action and face our fears, our feelings and beliefs can change based on these new experiences.

> Doing something that makes your child feel scared is essential for exposure therapy to work.

We also need to be clear that this is only Michael's first step toward overcoming his fear of dogs. Children learn to be afraid of things very quickly, which makes sense, since if something is truly dangerous, you may only have a few chances to learn to avoid it. On the flip side, we learn to embrace evidence of safety much more slowly, consistent with the better safe than sorry idea. For this reason, exposure therapy involves a lot of repetition.

Michael can't simply stay in the yard one day and then announce that he has triumphed over his anxiety. To overcome his fear, Michael needs to stay out in the yard on multiple occasions when the dog is outside. And then perhaps the next time the neighbor is outside Michael actually enters their yard and pets the dog. Eventually he may feed the dog a treat or help walk the dog around the block. And then, to fully master his fear of dogs, he will need to pet many different dogs in many different situations until he learns from his own experience that he can handle most dogs most of the time. To get there, he will need to practice, repeat, and practice some more.

When I'm working with families, I often find that at this point parents are relieved to have a potential solution for their child's anxiety, while their child may be more reluctant to start something that sounds so challenging. Focusing on facing fears head-on will be a different approach for your child, and it's natural if they are skeptical. Exposure therapy is not a new therapy though, and it has proven an effective treatment for decades. Before we move to learning how to do exposure therapy, we'll look briefly at how exposure therapy became a first-choice, effective treatment for childhood anxiety disorders and OCD.

## A BRIEF HISTORY OF EXPOSURE THERAPY

The earliest description of the use of exposure therapy for childhood fears harks back to Dr. Mary Cover Jones in 1924. Dr. Jones was an American psychologist whose trailblazing research with children earned her the informal standing as "the mother of behavior therapy." In her most famous study Dr. Jones tried seven different methods for removing preexisting fears in young children.

Many of the methods she tested are similar to things we often try as parents, such as waiting for a child's fear to pass on its own, explaining to our child that whatever it is they're scared of is not so bad, telling kids to get over it, employing distraction, and doing the feared activity ourselves to demonstrate that there is nothing to be afraid of.

Dr. Jones found that the straightforward method of having a child face his or her fears, which she called "negative adaptation without additional re-educative measures," successfully removed a child's fear, especially when a child was allowed to do something enjoyable, like eating candy, during the exposure.

She also found that having the frightened child observe other kids doing the activity without fear was helpful. Dr. Jones's interventions of almost 100 years ago still form the foundation for the use of rewards and modeling of brave behavior that we use today to engage children in exposure therapy.

The next wave of research into exposure therapy, ignited in the 1950s, further developed the techniques Dr. Jones had identified. Although not working specifically with children, Dr. Joseph Wolpe, a South African psychiatrist, conceived a process he called "systematic desensitization," whereby a patient is taught to relax while facing their fears. The goal, similar to Dr. Jones's technique of having children face their fear while eating a pleasurable food, was for the patient to gradually connect their feared object with a feeling of relaxation rather than one of feeling scared. Over time, research demonstrated that systematic desensitization was indeed effective and could work faster than talk therapy approaches.

In the 1960s, research by Dr. Albert Bandura, a prominent psychologist, demonstrated that kids could unlearn their fears by observing others. He demonstrated that kids like Michael who have a fear of dogs became less fearful after watching other children interact with dogs.

By the late 1960s and 1970s enough research had emerged supporting various treatments for anxiety that researchers began to compare them in an organized, controlled fashion. A couple of studies largely lost to history (perhaps because the researchers did not achieve the degree of renown as the others we have discussed) suggested that kids doing exposure by itself was more effective than watching other kids do the feared activity and that teaching kids to relax was not necessary for exposure to work.

The modern era of exposure therapy for childhood anxiety disorders was ushered in by Dr. Phil Kendall in the 1990s. His research expanded the use of treatment from the previous focus on specific phobias to children suffering from fears and worries related to separation, generalized anxiety, and social situations. He combined exposure exercises with relaxation techniques and strategies for problem-solving and changing anxiety-causing thinking patterns in a treatment called cognitive behavioral therapy, or CBT for short. Over time, CBT has been expanded to treat other childhood anxiety disorders, including OCD, panic disorder, and PTSD. Since Dr. Kendall's groundbreaking studies there have been over 100 clinical trials of CBT worldwide, making it by far the most studied treatment for childhood anxiety disorders. Exposure is the most important part of CBT.

With our brief tour of where exposure therapy comes from complete, let's look at how that history has led to our current understanding of what makes exposure therapy work.

## HOW DOES EXPOSURE THERAPY WORK?

Exposure therapy gives children like Michael the opportunity to learn that what they fear will happen rarely happens, and that they can handle feeling anxious until that feeling passes. This process gets easier with practice, both in the moment and over time, with repetition. Each additional episode of exposure to the feared situation builds more confidence and offers the child further proof that their anxiety is decreasing.

In terms of how this happens, one of the original theories suggested that exposure therapy works best if you replace a child's anxiety with a positive experience. This is why Dr. Jones paired exposure with pleasurable foods and snacks and Dr. Wolpe coached his patients how to relax during exposure. Rather than connecting a situation, place, or activity with feeling scared, children could instead connect the situation with positive feelings like relaxation or doing something enjoyable like eating a cookie, chocolate bar, or ice cream. The goal was to see these pairings rewire a formerly scary or terrifying situation to a new, positive association.

As early as the late 1960s there were signs coming from new research that you didn't necessarily need to pair exposures with a positive experience for them to be effective, and by the early 1980s, exposure appeared to work just as well all by itself, and the theory that a positive or calming emotion had to be used to replace anxiety lost scientific support.

Around the same time researchers became interested in the importance of thoughts and beliefs in anxiety treatment, the idea being that if mistakenly believing something to be dangerous leads to problems with anxiety, then treatment should focus on changing those beliefs. This theory led to the development of therapy techniques like CBT that help people recognize and change anxiety-causing thoughts. Recent research, including the treatment study my colleagues and I completed comparing parent-coached exposure therapy to CBT, suggests that kids learn best through exposure and that other therapy techniques are not needed and can actually make treatment less effective.

Until recently, something we call habituation has been the most dominant theory about how exposure therapy works. Habituation is the term for when you get used to something by doing it over and over again. That could be something that starts out causing anxiety, like a new job, but with each successive day at the office you get a little less anxious, until you're settled in and are confident in your new workplace and responsibilities. Habituation leads you to have less of an emotional reaction over time to a scenario that previously made you acutely, habitually nervous. We apply this logic to exposure therapy and have found that by doing an exposure over and over again, the volume of the anxious feelings eventually turns down.

Habituation is a helpful theory, but it doesn't explain some things, like why problems with anxiety sometimes come back after treatment. This and other unanswered questions led to the development of what anxiety researchers call inhibitory learning theory, the most up-to-date understanding of how exposure theory works.

This theory focuses on the expectations we have that connect feeling nervous to a situation. In the case of 16-year-old Maria, talking to people *connects* to feeling nervous because she *expects* people to laugh at her. What is new about inhibitory learning theory is that we don't unlearn the connection between talking and feeling nervous; it's always there. Instead, as Maria faces her fears, she accumulates new learning that begins to override the original connection between talking and feeling nervous. As a result, over time, the new connection between talking to people and feeling confident drowns out the nervous connection because it's been strengthened through repeated exposures during which other kids don't laugh at her. However, since the old connection between talking and feeling nervous was forged over years of suffering from anxiety, it has the potential to creep back on top of the more fragile new learning. This can often happen if a child is in a situation where they have a long history of feeling anxious but have not yet practiced facing their fear. Just because Maria has learned to be confident giving presentations in the therapist's office, where no children

Inhibitory learning theory suggests that to be most successful, exposures need to offer learning experiences that are as powerful as possible. One way we achieve this is by making exposures surprising. Exposures are most surprising, and therefore memorable, when a child is very afraid and certain something bad is going to happen but then it doesn't.

stare at her, doesn't necessarily mean she has learned to be confident presenting in a real-time school classroom packed with classmates.

Inhibitory learning theory suggests that to be most successful, exposures need to offer learning experiences that are as powerful as possible. One way we achieve this is by making exposures surprising. Exposures are most surprising, and therefore memorable, when a child is very afraid and certain something bad is going to happen but then it doesn't. That experiment adds up to offer a really strong learning experience that powerfully replaces old learning with new learning.

Most anxiety experts base their treatment on a combination of habituation and inhibitory learning theories. Despite some unanswered questions, the habituation theory brought us a long way, supporting decades of successful research and use of exposure to help kids with anxiety disorders. On the other hand, although inhibitory learning theory brings us closer to understanding how exposure works, it is a relatively new theory, and over time we will likely learn that it also does not have all the answers. For now, we have two well-tested theories for how exposure works. They have a lot of overlap and some important differences, but together they offer a solid foundation for how to help children face their fears most successfully and get better.

## OUR WORKING MODEL FOR EXPOSURE THERAPY

If parents are to trust me with the care of their children, I need to earn that trust by providing the best care possible. That's why we have based our approach at Mayo Clinic on history, theory, and research and then refined it over the years through our own clinical work and research. This process has led to a successful model that sets a foundation for how we use exposure therapy in our clinic.

Our goal for treatment is for children to no longer have problems resulting from feeling more nervous, worried, or scared than we would expect in reasonably safe situations. To have fewer problems with anxiety, kids need to feel less anxious. To feel less anxious, kids need to learn through their own experience that their fears are unlikely to come true.

At all times, underpinning our work is a primary goal to improve functioning through reducing, not getting rid of, a child's anxiety. As we saw earlier, feeling anxious is a normal part of life and not something we can or should remove completely.

As a result, treatment should help children learn they can handle their anxiety in a feared scenario and do things they need to do in their everyday lives despite those feelings. To prove successful, treatment needs to both help kids feel less anxious and improve their ability to do the things they need and want to do.

With those treatment goals in mind, we have four guiding principles to maximize the therapeutic power of exposure.

### Principle 1: Exposures need to be carried out frequently and intentionally

To help kids master their fears and worries we purposely and repeatedly do exposures. That means we don't wait for the feared scenario to happen but instead seek out opportunities to practice. To treat his fear of dogs, Michael can't simply wait for the neighbor's dog to come out. Instead, with a parent's help, he makes a plan to go over to the neighbors' house and pet their dog. Michael can't just do that once, he needs to repeat this action over and over, and then graduate up to making plans to go to his friends' houses and pet their family dogs, and then perhaps go to the local park to interact with the dogs there. Exposure therapy is an active treatment based on repeatedly setting up experiments to test one's fears.

### Principle 2: Exposures need to make children feel anxious

All theories on how exposures work agree that to be effective, exposure activities need to make children feel anxious. Whether the goal of an exposure is to learn that fear goes away over time or to allow for new learning to override old fears, neither of those will occur if the child does not go into the exposure feeling nervous. Reading a fun story about dogs with his mother will not be a helpful exposure if it doesn't make Michael fearful. When kids are feeling high levels of anxiety at the beginning of an exposure, it opens space for them to have a powerful learning experience when their fears don't come true. We don't shy away from challenging kids, and we don't do anything to reduce a child's fears and worries before the exposure begins. Using relaxation or distraction techniques to calm a child before beginning an exposure opens the risk of making the experience less authentic, surprising, convincing, or powerful.

### Principle 3: Exposures need to continue until children's fears are disproven

Exposure therapy experts agree that it's necessary to keep doing an experiment until the child learns something new. In our clinic, we view this learning as involving changes to beliefs and feelings. To be successful, an exposure needs to last until the child learns that what they are afraid of is unlikely to happen. Michael needs to keep petting his neighbor's dog until he realizes that it isn't going to bite him. Kids also need to continue an exposure until they learn that the anxiety they experience is manageable, which means Michael needs to keep petting the dog until he realizes that he can feel calm even if he is right next to the dog. If a child leaves a situation while they are still convinced something bad and unmanageable will happen, which is their typical response in daily life, they won't learn that the situation is actually safe. Moreover, during and after an exposure, it's important that the child does not do anything to prevent themselves from learning that the situation is reasonably safe. As we touched on earlier, efforts to avoid, seek reassurance, distract, or use rituals leave the child believing they were safe only because of what they did to prevent the feared outcome, rather than learning the situation was never inherently dangerous.

### Principle 4: Exposures need to be realistic

To be useful learning experiences, exposure activities need to be as close as possible to real-life situations to evoke authentic, credible feelings of anxiety. This means going to where the anxiety occurs. Michael can't simply pet his neighbor's dog or pet a single dog in a therapist's office. He needs to plan and do exposures to different dogs in different places. So if, as is usually the case, fears occur in many different ways and places, effective treatment needs to include completing exposures in all those ways and places.

---

At this point, with all four principles covered and fresh in your mind, you might be thinking, *That all makes sense, but what exactly am I supposed to be doing to help my child face their anxieties?* The goal for this chapter was to bring you to a place of feeling confident that responding to your child's anxiety by helping him or her face their fears is a long-established treatment. We're now going to delve into what exposure therapy looks like and how to turn the four guiding principles into concrete actions.

# 6

# The Different Types of Exposure

Now that we have introduced the theory behind exposure therapy, we are going to learn about what we specifically do during an exposure. We'll start off by introducing planned exposures, the foundation of therapy. Although we use planned exposures to treat all problems with anxiety, they will differ depending on what sets off a child's fears and worries. To that end, we will learn about three different types of exposures that you can do with your child. We'll wrap up this chapter with a discussion of how to transition from heavily structured planned exposures to more spontaneous and realistic *on-the-fly* exposures that apply what kids have learned to real-life situations.

## PLANNED EXPOSURES

Planned exposures are the core foundation of treatment for childhood anxiety disorders and, simply put, involve your child purposely doing something that makes them nervous for the sole purpose of learning through their own experience that this situation they've been so frightened of isn't so bad after all.

Planned exposures are set up with forethought and are designed to be the initial practice. You can think of planned exposures as being like your child going to soccer practice or a dance rehearsal. They offer a controlled and supportive environment where children and their families learn how to do exposures and where anxiety-provoking situations are first tackled. The goal of planned exposures is for your child to gradually learn that their fears are unlikely to come true and build confidence that they can handle these situations in daily life.

For Michael and his fear of dogs, his mother would make arrangements for the pair of them to go over to their neighbor's house on a calm Sunday afternoon when there will be plenty of time and they won't feel rushed. Before leaving their house, Michael and his mother would agree on a goal for the exposure, in this case to pet the dog with his mother standing right there beside him. At the same time as setting the goal, they would also write down what he is afraid will happen and how nervous he is about this. Michael and his mother would then go to the neighbor's house and, as planned, pet the dog for as long as needed until he learns that petting his neighbor's dog is not as dangerous as he thought and at no time does the dog bite him as feared.

Planned exposures are designed to maximize the general principles of effective exposures we learned in the last chapter: Exposures need to be frequent, intentionally cause anxiety, continue until fears are disproven, and be realistic.

Here is a list of the six main characteristics of successful planned exposures, to help make sure your child gets the most out of them.

## CHARACTERISTICS OF SUCCESSFUL PLANNED EXPOSURES

### Be intentional and consistent

Just as medications don't work if you don't take them as prescribed, exposures won't improve anxiety if you don't do them. This is arguably the most important point. Finding time to do planned exposures is fundamental to making progress. Michael and his mother can't simply wait for a dog to walk by; they need to take the initiative and plan a time to go over to the neighbor's house. If it's an option, working with a therapist can help by simply keeping you and your family accountable for completing planned exposures. But if you are carrying out exposures on your own, you will need to be intentional about adding exposures to your daily schedule.

### Go out and be active

Planned exposures require going to where the anxiety is. Frequently that means leaving the house. Michael and his mother need to go to his neighbor's house, his friends' houses, and the park. Maria, the 16-year-old with social anxiety we met earlier, needs to work with her parents to plan exposures to strike up conversations at figure-skating practice or talk to salesclerks at malls.

### Bring on anxiety

The goal of exposure therapy is to do something that makes your child nervous. Kids are learning that they can handle feeling anxious, do things even though it makes them feel uncomfortable, and that what they're afraid of doesn't actually happen. To achieve these outcomes, an exposure has to bring on anxiety or, for a child with OCD, perhaps disgust or a not-just-right sensation. This means planning activities that your child would not normally do, and may not want to do, simply because that activity will make a powerful exposure. A child afraid of contamination might go into a public bathroom and touch the stall door—not because they need to use the bathroom but because they believe it to be a source of germ contamination. Sometimes the activities we do for exposures are exaggerated to bring on anxiety more directly and not something we would typically do consciously, like rubbing a door handle and then rubbing our clothes.

### Rinse and repeat

Since kids learn to be safe in previously feared situations very slowly, planned exposures need to be done over and over again. That means each individual exposure needs to include layers of repetition. Michael can't merely walk over to the neighbor's house, pat the dog on its head, and go back home. Rather, he needs to sit there petting the dog over and over until he learns it is not going to bite or attack him. Planned exposures can be more challenging with social anxiety, which requires finding new people to talk to. So, with Maria, she and her parents can make an exposure repetitive by going into a store and asking where the sweatshirts are, and then going to another store and asking where the jeans are, and then to another store and asking if they sell hats, and so on. Repetition also involves planned exposures being repeated over time. Michael and his mother might organize two or three planned exposures at the neighbor's house before he feels comfortable around their dog and his new learning surpasses the old expectations. The number of required repetitions varies, and we will go into more detail about this when we put together specific exposure plans.

### Learn something new

Each exposure is set up to test the child's expectations that have made the safe situations seem scary. To do this successfully, exposure planning needs to be specific about what a child expects is going to happen. In Michael's case, he expects the dog will bite him. So, if he pets his neighbor's dog and the dog does not bite him, that is one piece of new learning that family dogs are typically safe. Or for 8-year-old Alex with separation anxiety, he might fear that if he is alone, he will get more and more upset until he can't handle it. But if he stays in his room alone, gets bored, and starts entertaining himself, he learns that being alone is not as overwhelming or bad as he expected. The amount of time it takes for kids to learn that a feared situation is safe depends on the exposure, and deciding when you can wrap up an exposure is one of the steps we will dive into later. Learning something new also means kids can't rely on rituals, avoidance, reassurance from parents, or other coping mechanisms during an exposure. All of those subtle forms of avoidance prevent kids from learning that they survived an exposure simply because it wasn't so bad, rather than because their parents helped them avoid or fix it.

### Be willing to do it again

The goal of each exposure is for a child to learn that it wasn't so bad and be willing to do it again. Planned exposures are practice to prepare kids and increase their confidence that they can handle situations that arise in everyday life without rituals or avoidance. We need to be clear from the beginning that we are not doing exposures just to complete them and check them off the list. Relief from anxiety does not occur because the exposure is over and your child never has to think about it again. The essence of planned exposures is that anxiety decreases because the child learned the situation was not as bad as they expected, despite the fact that they know they *will* be doing this again. At the end of petting his neighbor's dog, Michael needs to be able to say he is willing to go back the next day and do it all over again.

## THE THREE TYPES OF EXPOSURE

Now we know the basic components of a planned exposure, we're going to look at the different types of activities that can be done during exposures. Although planned exposures form the bedrock for the treatment of all anxiety disorders, the specific activity will depend on your child's fears. We learned earlier that there are three types of scenarios that can set off a child's anxiety and start the avoidance cycle: things in the world around them, thoughts in their heads, and feelings in their body. And so, we have three forms of exposure that address each of those types of fear. We're now going to look at each form of exposure so you can begin to think about which method is the best fit for your child's fears and worries.

### Action exposures (a.k.a. in vivo exposures)

Action exposures are designed to address fears and worries that are set off by things in the world, like meeting dogs, riding elevators, or talking to people. These are the most straightforward, powerful, and well-known types of exposure therapy. Action exposures are typically called *in vivo exposures,* which is a fancy way of saying exposures that are carried out in real life. Action-oriented, or in vivo, exposures are the most direct and experiential of the forms of exposure.

When children are afraid of a thing, place, or activity, they need to go there and do that thing until they learn it is not so dangerous. Michael petting the neighbor's dog is an action exposure, and so is Maria starting conversations with the other girls at ice skating practice. Other common action exposures include: giving speeches to a group, touching doorknobs and rubbing those germs on their

> Action-oriented, or in vivo, exposures are the most direct and experiential of the forms of exposure.

body, staying home alone while their parents walk around the block, purposely making a minor mistake on a homework assignment, walking upstream in a crowded hallway, watching videos of people throwing up, eating chewy food that a child fears will cause them to choke, standing on a balcony and looking over the edge, or holding a medical needle.

Although we will learn about two other forms of exposure, in general it is best to lead with action-oriented exposures whenever possible, because they are the most direct and powerful test of a child's fears. But sometimes there isn't a fitting action exposure to do or a tangible place to go to address a child's fears and worries, especially if they are worried about something that simply doesn't exist or isn't actually happening in the moment, which brings us to the next type of exposure.

### Thought exposures

When a child's anxiety is set off by thoughts in their head, for instance, worrying about the future, or scary memories of the past, or upsetting, intrusive OCD thoughts, then *thought or imaginal exposures* are the best treatment. In these situations, there isn't anything to go out and do in terms of action or activity because it's the thought itself that causes anxiety, regardless of what your child is doing or where they are.

The goal of thought exposures is for kids to learn that thoughts are just thoughts and cannot actually hurt them. To do this, kids will repeat their worry thought over and over and over until it gets boring. It turns out that if you repeat a thought over and over, no matter how unpleasant that thought is, it starts to lose its power and become boring, if not outright annoying.

When setting up a thought exposure, we have the child write down the scariest thought they have without making it positive. Kara, the 16-year-old with GAD, worries she will never get into college or get a good job, despite being a straight-A student and excelling in multiple activities. Her thought exposure might be to write down and then repeat out loud her main worry thought: *Because I failed the math test, I won't get into college and will never get a job.*

The key to understanding this thought exposure is that yes, it would be understandably upsetting to fail a test, not get into college, and never get a job. But most of us can think about that without getting overly anxious and having to overprepare and ask for reassurance.

So, Kara's goal for the thought exposure is to repeat, *Because I failed the math test, I won't get into college and will never get a job* over and over until her anxiety decreases. You will have noticed that Kara did not add anything like *But it probably won't happen because I usually do well,* because those types of statements, while in this case accurate, are attempts to avoid or rationalize away the worry.

To reduce the amount of worry and anxiety Kara experiences day to day, she needs to learn through thought exposures that she can handle having worry thoughts without doing anything to get rid of them.

In my experience, writing down the worry thought and then repeating it out loud, as Kara did, is the best way to start thought exposures. Repeating something aloud, no matter how horrible it is, soon gets boring, often pretty quickly, which is a powerful demonstration that thoughts are just thoughts. However, one potential pitfall of this is that some children find saying the upsetting thought out loud during a planned exposure therapy not entirely authentic, because in real life, the thoughts are of course happening in their heads and are silent to the outside world.

Another approach can be to have the child sit and silently repeat the thought in his or her head while imagining the distressing scenario happening. This method allows for more detail, including imagining pictures or images, and is often much more realistic and upsetting. These exposures can be more difficult, with anxiety decreasing more slowly, but with that they can also be more powerful. In our clinic, we typically encourage kids to first start by saying the thought out loud until it becomes boring. Then they can progress to exposures where they think about and picture the thought silently for several minutes and then repeat it aloud, going back and forth between these two approaches.

A third way to do thought exposures is for a child to write down the distressing thought. If the thought is only a single word, the child can sit and write that single word over and over again, until the thought of writing it one more time feels exasperating and repetitive to the point of total boredom. Or they may write a full sentence, a few sentences, a paragraph, or even more if they need to flesh out the fear. They can then reread what they have written and perhaps start saying it out loud.

Doing thought exposures is straightforward, but can seem a little strange at first. Parents are often concerned that repeating the distressing thought might make their child believe it more and might make things worse. They often wonder if it wouldn't be better to help their child understand that the thought is not true or repeat positive thoughts to build the child's confidence. And yes, it is always appropriate to *first* explain to the child why their fears and worries are unfounded and to reassure them that things will work out. But, when kids are suffering from anxiety despite repeated reassurance, not only has that reassurance not worked, it has become part of the avoidance cycle that maintains their fears. When working with families in our clinic, we encourage them to do thought exposures for the first time in a session with us to get the hang of it. To address concerns that repeating thoughts will make things worse, it may be helpful to know that there is a lot of research behind the value of thought exposure, deriving mostly from the study of OCD and PTSD.

With PTSD, people have experienced a traumatic event in the past and, long after that event, they continue to be plagued by overwhelmingly frightening and upsetting dreams, flashbacks, intrusive thoughts, and memories. This can happen after a person has been in a car accident, attacked, abused, the victim of a crime, or caught in a natural disaster. The problem is that although they are now safe, the thoughts, flashbacks, and memories of the traumatic event set off their anxiety and avoidance cycle in the present day. The most effective treatment for PTSD involves telling and retelling the story of that traumatic event over and over. The goal of this is to wear down those memories until they are no longer frightening or overwhelming. The memories of the event will never be pleasant because the event was traumatic, but the memories do not have to continue to be terrifying or overwhelming. When treating PTSD, these types of thought exposures are often called prolonged exposure therapy or narrative exposure and can be very effective.

As with PTSD, there is a long history of using thought exposures with OCD. Children with OCD may have intrusive thoughts about things that would be very frightening or upsetting if they actually occurred, like Hector's fears that he was stabbing someone just by pointing a body part at them. Although stabbing someone would obviously be lethal or fatal, as well as a criminal act, the thought of it happening is not. Hector needs to learn through exposure that thinking about stabbing people is unpleasant, but the thought doesn't make him actually do it, nor do thoughts hurt him or anyone else. Of course, this treatment needs to be undertaken only after OCD is correctly diagnosed and is not appropriate for a child who has thoughts of hurting people because they are angry or have a history of violence.

Hector therefore might start his exposures by repeating, *I'm going to stab my mother,* over and over until the thought gets boring and he comes to realize he can have these upsetting thoughts without acting on them or getting overwhelmed. As mentioned earlier, Hector's thoughts mostly bother him when a body part is pointing at someone. So, the next exposure might be for him to point his knee at his mother while repeating, *I am stabbing my mother.* This is a good example of combining an action exposure—pointing his knee at his mother—with a thought exposure—repeating *I am stabbing my mother.*

When deciding whether to use a thought exposure or action exposure or a combination, it is best to consider how to most directly help your child bring on their anxiety. This usually means if there is some action that brings on anxiety, we should include that in the exposure. Even when thoughts are the most direct cause of the anxiety, as in the examples above, adding in an action often makes the exposure more realistic, heightening the anxiety and creating a more powerful learning experience. So, Hector points his knee at his mother to bring on more frightening thoughts of stabbing her or Kara can repeat her worry thought about getting poor grades while doing math homework quickly and intentionally not rechecking her answers.

Thought exposures can also be used to make action exposures more focused and powerful. Take Alex, the 8-year-old boy afraid of separation, who panics when his mother drops him off at school and later follows her around the house all evening. To give Alex the chance to learn that he can handle being alone even if he has scary thoughts, his exposures might involve sitting in a room alone—an action exposure—while repeating *Mom is never coming back* over and over again—a thought exposure.

Leading up to this activity, Alex and his parents would have prepared for this combined exposure by first separately doing action exposures—by having him be in a room alone—and also thought exposures—by having Alex repeat worry thoughts with his parent next to him. Through single and combined exposures, Alex learns that not only can he handle being at home without his parents but he can also independently handle having upsetting thoughts about their absence.

It should also be said that thoughts, worries, and memories that cause kids distress can also be very upsetting for parents. Worries about the future can be a little too close to our own worries for our children, intrusive OCD thoughts can involve violent or sexual themes that we would prefer our children did not think about, and PTSD memories can be traumatic for everyone involved.

Having your child repeat those thoughts out loud doesn't only make us uncomfortable but may lead us to question if this is truly the right solution. My perspective is that if a child is already having these thoughts, then there is no undoing it. And if that thought is haunting them by frequently popping up and distressing them, trying to push it away or ignore it will only make matters worse. The best way to relieve their distress is to drain the fear and anxiety out of the thought through exposure.

### Bodily sensation exposures

The third major form of exposure is called interoceptive exposure. This form of exposure is all about intentionally re-creating and bringing on the physical or bodily symptoms of panic and anxiety. We lead with interoceptive exposures when a child's fear centers on experiencing physical feelings and sensations, for example, if they are afraid of having panic attacks or worry stomachaches will lead to vomiting. The goal of interoceptive exposures is for kids to learn that even if the physical symptoms of anxiety and panic are unpleasant and uncomfortable, they are not dangerous. And that kids can walk around, talk, be in crowds, give a presentation, or do math problems while feeling anxious and panicky.

Exposures to bodily sensations were developed for and are used most commonly to treat panic disorder. Think of Nora, the 14-year-old, generally well-adjusted teenager whose panic attacks were increasingly keeping her homebound. We understand panic disorder to be in essence a fear of fear, that is, when Nora's heart rate increases or her chest tightens slightly, it leads to an automatic fear reaction that includes more heart racing and chest tightening in addition to dizziness, shakiness, and inability to catch her breath. Not only are these feelings even more frightening, but they make her extremely self-conscious, because she is also certain that her classmates can tell something is wrong with her.

To feel better, Nora needs to break the connection between the initial heart racing and chest tightening with the resulting fear and escalating physical symptoms. To do this, we would purposely bring on the panic feelings through interoceptive exposures like hyperventilating, breathing through a cocktail straw, running up and down stairs, or spinning in a chair. If Nora experiences these symptoms over and over without losing control, passing out, or experiencing some other dreaded outcome, then she will come to learn that the physical experiences associated with panic are merely unpleasant rather than outright frightening.

Hyperventilation is one of the best ways to bring on the overall physical experience of panic and anxiety. At our clinic, we coach a child to breathe deeply without pauses, deeper than usual and at just a bit quicker rate than we'd normally breathe but not fast. If anybody does this for a while, soon enough they will feel dizzy, light-headed, out of breath, experience tingly sensations, and become very aware of their heart racing, feelings similar to a panic attack. When kids are specifically nervous about running out of air or not being able to breathe, breathing through a small, narrow cocktail straw is a powerful way to re-create that experience. Other interoceptive exposures include running up and down the stairs to get the heart pounding or spinning in a swivel chair to feel dizzy.

We typically begin exposures to bodily sensations by having kids first do the activity for five seconds to try it out. Five seconds of one of these exercises won't make them feel too uncomfortable but is a chance to make sure they are doing it right and they are on board with the exercise. We then build on that and do it for longer—around 15 seconds the second time. And then keep working up incrementally from 15 seconds to 30 seconds, 30 seconds to 45 seconds, all the way up to a full minute. We then stay at a minute and repeat. The goal is for the child to be able to say that, although they felt very uncomfortable, they no longer feared that they would panic or pass out or that anything bad would happen.

In addition to panic disorder, interoceptive exposures can be used for other fears and worries about bodily sensations. An otherwise healthy boy who worries about having a heart attack might do interoceptive exposures by running up and down stairs to learn that it is safe for his heart to pound. And Maria might run up and down the stairs to look flushed and out of breath before giving a speech to learn that her peers don't seem to notice or care if she looks nervous.

Bodily sensation exposures can also be combined with action-oriented and thought exposures. When working with children who have panic disorder, step one is for them to learn that they can handle physical symptoms of panic through hyperventilating in a therapist's office. Next, they need to learn that they can handle these feelings while out and about, so we might have them hyperventilate and then walk around in public spaces, or start a conversation, or, if in our clinic, we might have them do math problems on the board in front of the therapy group.

As with all exposures for anxiety disorders, the activities we have kids do are reasonably safe. With bodily sensation exposures this includes ensuring that a child does not have any health conditions that would prevent them from doing the physical exercises to bring on panic feelings.

---

Now that we have covered the three forms of exposure that we use to treat the three sources that set off fears and worries, let's look at how to transition from highly controlled, planned exposures to handling feared situations in everyday life.

## ON-THE-FLY EXPOSURES

Planned exposures, whether carried out with actions, thoughts, or physical sensations, are structured practice to build confidence. The goal is for kids to be willing and able to face these or similar feared situations when they arise in everyday life. By their very nature of being thoughtfully prepared for, planned exposures may lack some of the realism necessary for maximum effectiveness. For that reason, after we have had initial success with planned exposures, we transition to what we call *on-the-fly exposures* in everyday life situations. As the name suggests, on-the-fly exposures are carried out spontaneously in the moment when a child is confronted with an actual feared situation.

Let's say socially anxious Maria has worked through a number of planned exposures to speaking in public. She and her father have successfully gone to the mall and moved from store to store asking questions of salesclerks. Then, one evening, the family is at a restaurant having dinner, and Maria becomes nervous that she will look foolish ordering her food. Rather than Mom or Dad ordering for her, as they did in the past, they remind her this is an excellent chance for an on-the-fly exposure. Together, they identify what she fears will happen—that she'll mumble and be asked to repeat herself, which will make her blush and want the ground to open up and swallow her whole—and see how she can turn this into an exposure by not only ordering her own food but also asking the waitress which desserts she recommends. Maria orders steak, fries, salad, and lemonade and asks about dessert. After the waitress has left their table, she and her parents review how it went. She felt shaky doing the exposure, but it went okay, and she realized that nothing happened that she couldn't handle.

The basic goal of planned and on-the-fly exposures is the same: to learn that the feared situation isn't so bad after all. The biggest difference is that on-the-fly exposures occur naturally in the moment, rather than being activities specifically designed to bring on anxiety, as with planned exposures.

By definition, on-the-fly exposures are more realistic, as they are real-life situations, and often elicit higher levels of anxiety than planned exposures. While on-the-fly exposures more successfully achieve realism, they typically do not involve the continued repetition until anxiety decreases that can be achieved with planned exposures. Although Maria could certainly push herself to talk to the waitress when she returns to ask how the meal is going, it would be impractical to keep asking question after question until her anxiety decreased.

For Michael and his fear of dogs, on-the-fly exposures might include approaching a family at the park and asking to pet their dog. Again, this is a relatively quick exposure that does not involve much planning and it wouldn't be repeated, as it wouldn't be practical to ask a stranger to hang around for 20 minutes until Michael feels confident that their dog won't bite him and allows his anxiety to decrease before walking away.

On-the-fly exposures can, despite the name, be prepared for ahead of time. Michael's mother could mention that if they see a dog at the park that afternoon it would be a good opportunity for an on-the-fly exposure. On-the-fly exposures can also include some repetition; Maria might push herself to ask the waitress questions at three separate times during the meal. Most important, on-the-fly exposures are a step between planned exposures and living life without avoiding fear. They involve less structure, support, and review, and they offer more spontaneity and realism. You can think of planned exposures as the initial heavy lifting and on-the-fly exposures as the fine-tuning that comes after. Together, they add up to make a complete treatment package.

---

Action, thought, and bodily sensation exposures, both planned and on the fly, form the foundation of our treatment of anxiety and OCD. Before we put together a step-by-step plan for how to set up, do, and end exposures, we're going to look at the central and incredibly important role that you as parents play during exposure therapy.

# 7

# The Role of Parents

As a parent, guardian, or caregiver, you play an essential role in the treatment of your child's anxiety. Exposure therapy is hard work, and central to our program is a belief that all children will be more successful if they have an exposure coach at home to support them. In this chapter, we're going to outline what you can do to help your child successfully master anxiety and OCD. Parents' roles certainly change as kids get older, and with different levels of child cooperation, but all parents will likely benefit from being aware of the concepts discussed in this chapter to help exposure therapy be successful.

As a parent, guardian, or caregiver, you play an essential role in the treatment of your child's anxiety. Exposure therapy is hard work, and central to our program is a belief that all children will be more successful if they have an exposure coach at home to support them.

Treatment in our clinic is based on the idea that parents are an essential part of the process. And this is true from the very start, when parents identify that something is going on with their child that might need to be addressed. I could probably count on one hand the number of times families have said that the child asked to see a therapist. The vast majority of the time, parents notice the problem and decide to seek help on their child's behalf. To me, this illustrates how fundamental a parent's perspective is to treatment.

This means that parents' opinions and insights need to be included when deciding if a child's symptoms are an anxiety disorder, applying the avoidance cycle to a child's experience, or planning an exposure. Of course, we need to include and listen to the child's perspective of their own experience too, but typically the parent's perspective is just as important. This is not surprising with young children, since we would not expect a 7-year-old to have the ability to accurately recall their feelings and behavior and judge the degree to which it differs from that of their peers.

The same can also be true of teenagers, who may feel embarrassed or overwhelmed by their anxiety and prefer to downplay its importance or impact on their lives. In those cases, even though parents may have limited opportunities to observe their teen in the moment, such as during social interactions, parents often recognize the signs of isolation, withdrawal, and avoidance of activities as well as their impact on their teen's well-being.

The bottom line is this: Your perspective as a parent is important, and you play an important role in gathering information about your child's anxiety. If you think something is a problem or sets off your child's anxiety, make sure it gets added to the exposure plan, even if your child disagrees.

## BECOMING AN EXPOSURE COACH

An essential role for parents is to give their child warm support and encouragement. As parents we know and embrace this, but we also know that parenting is hard and we sometimes get stressed, irritated, and overwhelmed ourselves. This is especially true when our child's anxiety makes daily life harder and causes us to worry about their future. It's challenging to provide calm support when we are nervous that our child won't be able to handle an exposure and have a nagging doubt that it might make things worse. And if you get frustrated doing exposures, your child may pick up on it and get frustrated too, and the process can be quickly derailed. Our goal as parents is to do our best to remain calm, warm, and supportive and serve as our child's cheerleader.

We opened this chapter reminding ourselves that exposure therapy is hard work. Most likely, kids, especially younger ones, are going to need parental help and guidance understanding what an anxiety disorder is, figuring out how it applies to them, and making a plan to fix things. Part of your job will involve helping them along. Even if you are working with a therapist, you will probably meet with that person at most one hour a week. That leaves a lot of time where you are the main source of support. At our clinic, we always work with kids and parents together for the entire session, all the time. So, if you are able to find a therapist to work with, I encourage you to ask to be involved in your child's care.

Keeping in mind this commitment to being active, warm, and supportive, a parent's new defined role in our anxiety treatment is as an exposure coach. On the first day of our treatment program, I explain to families that it is our responsibility as therapists to help them, kids and parents, do exposures during appointments, so they can learn firsthand how to do them. And then it is the parents' responsibility to help kids do exposures between appointments. Eventually, it's the child's responsibility to do exposures on their own, but parents actively coach their kids through exposures until kids can do them independently.

## THE MOTIVATION PLAN

If you are going to be responsible for making sure exposures get done, then you are going to need some tools to do that. We already know that exposure therapy is hard work and mastering anxiety or OCD can take a lot of practice. Add on top of that, the prospect of feeling better in a couple months is lousy motivation for working hard right here, right now. We can pretty much guarantee there will be times when your child won't want to cooperate. At our clinic, we follow four strategies we call the motivation plan, that parents can use to help kids stay motivated. As always, the way we do each of these looks different for a 7-year-old versus a 17-year-old, but the principles are the same.

### Small steps

If Michael's mother were to hear the explanation of exposure therapy and say, *I get it. Michael simply needs to face his fear. I'll take him to the dog park, throw him in, and he can come out when he is no longer afraid of dogs,* it would not go well. Michael would be terrified, argue with his mother, and not be open to any new learning. Instead, he and his mother need to make a plan to start easy and take small steps. Kids generally make the best progress when each exposure pushes them to do something a bit harder than the exposure before. When activities become too hard or move too quickly, kids are more likely to push back, get stuck, and stop making progress.

Ideally, parents and kids work together in small steps. This can be done in two ways. First off, we make a treatment plan, often called a fear ladder, which is a list of ways to face a particular fear. It starts easy and gradually gets more challenging; in the next chapter we'll learn how to draw one up. Second, each exposure is planned together. This is usually somewhat of a compromise. Parents are often excited about their child overcoming anxiety and returning to normal life, so they want to progress as fast as possible. Kids on the other hand are often feeling nervous and want to take things slow. Our goal is to find a pace that parents can be patient with and kids can accept.

When planning exposures, remember to balance being warm and accepting with being firm and active. Exposure therapy goes most smoothly when we let kids take the lead, making a list of activities to work on and choosing a next step that feels manageable. However, we are not helping our child if we sit passively by while they leave out important fears, don't make a decision, or choose the same activity over and over without progressing. So, in the end, parents are in charge of making sure a complete fear ladder has been drawn up and that it captures all the fears that need to be addressed. If kids can't or won't decide what to do for the next exposure, you as the parent must take the lead and decide for them.

## Praise and ignoring

Our attention as parents is an important part of the avoidance cycle that keeps kids stuck in anxiety and also a powerful tool for treatment. When kids are anxious or upset, they look to us for help. That's a natural human response. When our kids are anxious, we as parents love to swoop in and fix things, which is also a natural human response. However, when a child's fear has blown up into an anxiety disorder, then parents soothing and fixing things becomes a form of avoidance that maintains anxiety and distress. And if parents don't respond quickly enough when kids are anxious, kids will typically ramp up their anxious reaction until they succeed in convincing us that they need our help. Over time, this can lead to kids acting more and more anxious as they understand it is the most effective way to receive our assistance.

As a rule of thumb, if you pay attention and help your child, whatever your child did to get that help, they will do it again. If your child gets help when they appear overwhelmed with anxiety, they will become overwhelmed with anxiety to signal that they need help. If your child gets your help when they are calmly trying to face their fears, then they will do so again in the future.

One of our jobs as parents is to use attention and support to encourage calm cooperation. When your child is working with you, picking an activity for an exposure, and cooperating with that exposure, give lots of warm support, affection, and encouragement. However, if your child is acting overwhelmed by anxiety and whining, complaining, being obstructive, or getting angry, it is best for you to walk away until your child is ready to cooperate.

Removing attention because your child is not cooperating when they are clearly anxious and upset is really hard to do. That's why we start with small steps. If you feel confident that you have done your best to identify a small, manageable step, it makes it a little bit easier to walk away, especially if you remind yourself that as soon as your child is ready to work, you will give them your full warmth, support, and attention.

### Set goals and reward progress

With the true payoff from exposure therapy often waiting months down the road, it helps if parents work with their children to create a plan of short-term goals and rewards for success. These goals should focus on things under the child's control, primarily cooperating and completing exposures. Your child can't control how they feel, and they can't make themselves feel calm in a feared situation, so we should avoid goals such as *we will go on a shopping trip when you are no longer afraid to order your own food.* Rather, set goals such as doing 5 or 10 exposures. With younger kids this can be set up like a traditional reward system. Every time they do an exposure, they earn a point, and you can set levels of points to do fun things, like get ice cream, stay up later than normal bedtime, go to a basketball game, pick a prize, or take a trip to the zoo. With teenagers, it might go over better to approach it collaboratively like SMART goal setting. This is more self-driven and involves setting personal goals that are Specific, Measurable, Achievable, Relevant, and Time-bound. In the end, the goal of either approach is to reward your child's hard work and celebrate progress.

### Consequences

The fourth component of the motivation plan is to bring in mild consequences when your child refuses to do an exposure. Exposures should be treated like schoolwork: If kids haven't finished their homework, fun activities like TV, gaming, and friends are placed on hold until the homework is done. Similarly, if your child hasn't completed an exposure, then they lose access to electronics, seeing friends, or other fun activities until the exposure is done. If you remind your child it is time for an exposure and they angrily refuse, rather than engaging in arguing or negotiating, you should ignore them and remove your attention. However, if once you walk away they start playing video games, the exposure will never get done. So, in addition to not arguing you can remind them, *It is your choice to not do the exposure, but remember there are no fun activities until it is done.* Then you walk away, they get bored and figure out they should do the exposure to have their privileges returned; they do the exposure and your day gets back on track. This is a lot easier said than done, and it is fair to say that we spend a good amount of our time in the clinic helping parents put a motivation plan in place.

Parents can also use what I like to call therapeutic consequences. These fit nicely when kids have advanced to doing on-the-fly exposures.

A therapeutic consequence means that if a child refuses to do a reasonable exposure, they will be expected to complete two planned exposures at a later time. So, if Maria refuses to order her food at the restaurant for fear of making a mistake and insists on reverting to her parents doing it for her, she will be required to call restaurants and ask what time they close as a first exposure and then undertake a second exposure of asking directions in public.

Therapeutic consequences serve two purposes. If the situation is actually too hard, then the child can benefit from additional exposure practice to reduce anxiety and build confidence for the next time they are in that situation. And also, if kids are deciding to be resistant, the prospect of two exposures rather than one can help them make a better choice in the moment.

---

Your motivation plan will likely include each of these four aspects. Once the plan is in place, if your child is reluctant to complete the next small step of an exposure, you can remind them of their progress toward their next reward and that they will experience a consequence for refusal until the exposure is complete. This allows you to remove attention from resistant behavior and let the prospect of a consequence convince the child to cooperate, rather than resorting to arguing or pleading with your child.

## COACHING INDEPENDENCE

The final important role you as a parent will play is helping translate what kids learn from doing specific exposures into everyday life. This involves two main points. First, as kids learn through exposure that their fears are unfounded, they then need to use that knowledge to approach life rather than avoiding it. Transitioning from planned exposures to on-the-fly exposures is part of this journey. This process is less structured and involves a new mindset that says, *Yes, I will continue to feel scared, nervous, and worried at times; and this is an opportunity to face my fears.* You will play an important part in helping your child gradually adopt this perspective by gentle reminders, support, and coaching them to face their fears spontaneously when anxiety arises during daily life.

The second lesson is for you, and it is the realization that your child can indeed face their fears and manage their anxiety independently. You will learn this through your own experience of watching your child successfully complete exposures as well as through walking away from your child and letting them handle anxiety and frustration independently. You begin to learn this during controlled, planned exposures and then eventually by watching your child be successful on the fly in real-world situations.

When you as a parent do things and fix things to shield your child from anxiety, we call it accommodation. Accommodation might be Michael's mother going into the neighbors' yard to fetch his ball because he is afraid the dog might come out. Or Maria's parents ordering food for her at the restaurant. Or Alex's parents never going on a date because he is afraid to stay with a sitter. Or Aaron's parents climbing the stairs to the 12th floor of their hotel to avoid the elevators. In each of these examples, the parents are simply taking care of their kids and just trying to get through the moment. We have to keep life going. But, over time parental accommodation robs kids of the chance to learn they can handle feared situations on their own. A shortcut may save the moment, but it won't fix the future.

To combat our naturally ingrained desire to fix things for our kids, parents need to consciously apply the skills they practice during planned exposures to everyday life. That means if your child is overly anxious in a situation, encourage them to face their fears. If a situation is too hard, help them break it down into smaller steps, rather than completely avoid it. You can use attention, rewards, and consequences to help motivate them as needed. And, if anxiety wins in the moment and you have to make an accommodation to help them keep going, make sure there is a therapeutic consequence to help them be successful the next time.

## WHAT ABOUT THE REST OF LIFE?

Parents are often interested in how other factors may affect their child's anxiety, interfere with exposure therapy, and what else they can do to help their kids grow up healthy and resilient. When kids have an anxiety disorder or OCD, exposure therapy is the central aspect of treatment. However, other elements of healthy living provide an important foundation. Everything is worse, including anxiety and OCD, when kids are tired, stressed, or have too much pent-up energy. Getting exercise, adequate sleep, and healthy eating sets kids up to feel better and be more successful with exposure and life in general.

Other life stressors can make anxiety worse and exposures harder to implement. Kids today have new digital opportunities and challenges that can be simultaneously exciting and overwhelming. Too much screen time, whether gaming, surfing social media, or watching videos, can crowd out physical activity and in-person interactions, which can make kids feel more restless, irritable, and anxious. Connecting with peers through social media has replaced the phone cord stretched across the living room as a staple of teen life. However, the constant need to manage one's online presence, seek others' approval, and not miss out on what everyone else is doing can be exhausting over time. Parents should feel warranted limiting screen time and attempting to make sure their child's online experience is healthy.

I also encourage parents to look after their own well-being. Coaching your child through exposure therapy for anxiety and OCD is a stressful addition to already busy lives. Parents often ask how they can implement the plan we have created during daily life, where the family is home together for only a few hours in the evening after school, when kids have siblings who deserve time and attention, or kids split time between divorced parents' homes.

I encourage parents to prioritize and do what works for them as parents. In terms of priorities, just because your child is experiencing anxiety does not mean that right now is the best time to work on it. Maybe family life is too busy or there are other, bigger fires to put out now. In that case, we make a plan to return our attention to the child's anxiety in the future. We are not ignoring it, we will work on it, but not right now. In terms of doing what works with siblings, some parents decide that it is easiest to have their child with anxiety and their siblings all do exposures or equivalent challenging tasks, to keep everything even and so no one feels left out. Some parents enlist a responsible older sibling to assist with exposures, while others decide it works best to explain to the siblings they will need to be patient as parents work through anxiety with their brother or sister.

Sharing the load between parents and supporting each other can go a long way toward making exposure coaching more rewarding. Collaboration can be more challenging across multiple households. Over the years, we have had many divorced parents go through our program. Some are interested in working together. Other times we only meet one parent or parents rotate appointments. There is no one-size-fits-all solution, so we work with parents to find a plan they feel most comfortable with and then revise that plan as needed.

---

This chapter covered how you as a parent can coach your child through exposure therapy to successfully master their anxiety and OCD. Having worked with families for 20 years and being a parent myself, I know everything in this chapter is easier said than done. I tell parents that exposure therapy is hard for kids because they have to face their fears. But it is also hard for parents, who not only have to face their own fears of their child not succeeding but, on top of that, feel the helplessness of not being allowed to jump in and fix a situation for their kids. As a parent, it can at times be a rotten way to feel, but I assure you that when kids rise to the occasion and make progress, the relief and pride you will feel as parents is worth all the struggle. Just as kids learn how to do exposures through practice, parents learn how to best coach exposures through direct experience.

Now that we have all the basic principles of exposures and coaching laid out, we can put them all together in a concrete plan to help your child face their fears.

# 8

# A Step-by-Step Guide to Exposure Therapy

It's now time to put all the knowledge we've covered into practice with a step-by-step guide for preparing, planning, and doing exposures. We'll start off by using the avoidance cycle to guide an exposure plan that addresses your child's individual needs. Then we'll make a list of specific exposure activities to do, and finally, we'll detail how to set up, do, and learn from exposures. The goal for this chapter is for you as a parent to feel confident that you know how to go about helping your child face their fears. The chapters in the final section of this book will tailor these steps specifically to the different types of anxiety disorders and OCD.

## STEP 1: BUILDING FROM THE AVOIDANCE CYCLE

The avoidance cycle we looked at in Part 1 to help understand your child's anxiety or OCD now provides the foundation for building an exposure plan tailored to your child. We begin creating this by listing the items that set off your child's anxiety, whether they are situations and activities, thoughts and worries, and/or feelings in their body. For each of the items that set off anxiety, we will need to plan exposures that include a combination of going there and doing that, or repeating that thought, or bringing on those panic feelings. As you'll see below, we need a thorough list of all the situations, thoughts, and feelings that set off your child's anxiety, because if we miss some important ones there's a good chance those fears and worries will stick around.

> The avoidance cycle we looked at in Part 1 to help understand your child's anxiety or OCD now provides the foundation for building an exposure plan tailored to your child.

Next, we need to identify the expectations your child has that make safe situations seem scary. We'll draw on those expectations to turn exposures into experiments. Exposure therapy will help your child rewire those anxiety-causing expectations through their own experiences. We learned earlier that exposures are experiments, and those experiments need to be focused on testing and disproving the expectations that make safe situations, thoughts, or feelings scary for your child.

Lastly, we need to list the ways your child avoids feared situations to be alert for behaviors that will prevent new learning from happening. Since avoidance maintains anxiety, if your child does any form of partial avoidance, or seeks reassurance, or does a ritual during or after an exposure, it can prevent them from learning that the situation is safe. Specifically, they will go away believing that nothing bad happened during the exposure because of their avoidance, rituals, or reliance on parents, rather than because the activity was simply not dangerous. For exposures to be effective experiments, you as the parent need to help your child resist doing any avoidance, reassurance seeking, or rituals.

Once you and your child feel confident that you understand how your child's anxiety fits into the avoidance cycle, you'll be ready to start making lists of exposures to do.

## STEP 2: BUILDING A FEAR LADDER

The list of activities we draw up to use for exposures is called a fear ladder. The idea is that we break down facing your child's fear into steps and stack them in order—starting with the easiest and climbing up to more challenging exposures. In their graded construction, fear ladders begin to implement the first component of our motivation plan: take small steps.

Fear ladders also provide structure by outlining a general plan to follow. When it's time to do an exposure, you and your child don't have to brainstorm the next activity from scratch, you can simply look at your fear ladder and pick one. Fear ladders also help us to be thorough. If you have identified all the ways life sets off your child's anxiety, you are less likely to miss working on something important. Finally, fear ladders can be a way to track progress. You can cross steps off your ladder as you master them and tangibly see what is being accomplished, day by day, week by week. As with any list, we feel accomplishment when we get to check off items.

You can begin the process of making a fear ladder by reviewing the items from your child's avoidance cycle that set off their anxiety. If your child has more than one type of anxiety, for instance, social anxiety and an OCD fear of germs, I recommend you make a separate fear ladder for each.

Once you and your child have picked a fear to work on, make a list of all the ways, in what situations, and during what activities that fear comes up. Then take each of the items from the list and turn it into an exposure activity. Think about whether this sort of fear or worry would be best tackled through an action exposure, thought exposure, or bodily sensation exposure. Remember, action exposures are always going to be the go-to and the most powerful, so if there is a place to go or activity to do that sets off anxiety, do that for the exposure. Finally, take your list of exposures and put it in order from easiest to hardest.

To give you a working example, here's a fear ladder that Michael and his parents might make together so they can work on his fear of dogs.

### Michael's fear ladder

1. Watch videos of dogs barking
2. Stand on the front lawn and watch the neighbor's dog across the street
3. Arrange with the neighbor to go over and stand close to his dog while it's on the leash
4. Arrange with the neighbor to go over and pet the neighbor's dog
5. Walk the neighbor's dog on a leash
6. Play fetch with the neighbor's dog
7. Go to a friend or family member's house and pet their dog
8. Go to the Humane Society and pet dogs of different ages and sizes one at a time
9. Ask a stranger at the park if you can pet their dog
10. Pet dogs of all sizes at the dog park with a parent

As you can see, Michael's fear ladder starts with something easy—watching dog videos—which makes Michael only a little uncomfortable. Then he gradually works his way up to interacting directly and independently with different dogs. When doing these exposures, Michael and his parents work with a dog they know to be safe, as it would not be reasonable or appropriate for a child to walk up to and pet unfamiliar dogs. Finally, Michael completes his fear ladder with the biggest challenge—petting dogs at a dog park.

Michael's fear ladder illustrates the three components of a successful fear ladder:

1. Start off with something easy that doesn't cause your child much anxiety. This will be an exposure your child is willing to start with because it's not too challenging. The goal of the first exposure is more to learn how to do exposures and have an initial success rather than to tackle a significant fear.
2. Complete the fear ladder with an exposure that is extra challenging and involves your child facing their greatest fear. Try to come up with a scenario even more frightening than what your child experiences in daily life so they can *overlearn* that their anxiety is misleading them. Accomplishing this ultimate, major exposure sends a strong message to the child that they can handle just about anything that anxiety throws at them. As always, even though the exposure is very challenging, it is still a reasonably safe activity that does not involve more risk than normal daily life.
3. Be mindful to include enough items in between the starting and closing items to make sure you don't miss any important situations that set off your child's anxiety or OCD.
   Make sure you have an exposure item for all the different situations, activities, thoughts, or bodily sensations that set off your child's fear. This is where the principle of small steps comes in. We would like to have enough items on our fear ladder to get from the easiest item to the most challenging by taking a series of small confidence-building steps.

Over the years I have learned that making fear ladders is challenging and takes a lot of practice. The upcoming chapters in Part 3 include specific directions and examples for building fear ladders to address the different anxiety disorders to help you get started.

Once you and your child have created a fear ladder, you'll be ready to start doing actual exposures.

## STEP 3: SETTING UP AN EXPOSURE

Planned exposures require kids and parents to work together to decide what activity to do and to be clear about what they hope to learn from the exposure. Before doing each planned exposure, I recommend you and your child take a few minutes to sit down and set things up together. In our clinic we have families record all their planned exposures on a paper form, and we have included a worksheet in the appendix at the back of this book, should you wish to use it. Filling out an exposure form not only helps a family follow all the steps to get the most out of an exposure, but it also creates a record in black and white of hard work and success.

### Pick an activity

You and your child begin an exposure by choosing the activity to complete. Use your fear ladder to guide your selection of an activity that is a small step forward. You may need to revise an activity from the fear ladder or create a new one if the next step is too challenging and would work better broken up into two bite-size exposures instead. To avoid disagreements during the exposure, make sure your child understands what they need to do to successfully complete the activity. Although it is best for kids and parents to pick an exposure activity together, remember that you as the parent are responsible for keeping things on track and you are the final judge as to whether each exposure activity stands up as an adequate step forward. Once more using Michael as an example, he and his mother might set up an exposure to go to the neighbor's house and stand in the hall while the neighbor holds the dog on the leash in the living room.

### Make it an experiment

We're not doing exposures simply to make your child uncomfortable and life difficult. We're doing them to test the accuracy of your child's expectations that something bad will happen that they can't handle. This comes back to the avoidance cycle and challenging the expectations that make safe situations seem dangerous. Is your child afraid of something bad happening? If so, what? Or are they afraid that they won't be able to handle their anxiety on their own?

As part of setting an exposure as a proper experiment, your child needs to specify what they fear will happen. You want to be as specific as possible. So, when Michael and his parents are setting up an exposure to be near his neighbor's dog, he needs to be clear with his parents that he expects the neighbor's dog will run over and bite him. The reason for clearly specifying what Michael expects will happen is that when he does the exposure and the dog does not bite him, he now has one piece of evidence that contradicts his expectations. This new evidence starts the process of building learning that makes him feel a little more confident to move on and do the next exposure.

At this point you may be thinking, *But how do we set up an exposure as an experiment if my child doesn't expect anything bad to happen; they just think it is scary and they don't want to do it?*

In that case, you can frame the exposure with your child as an experiment to test their expectation that the activity will be too overwhelming to handle. If Kara plans an exposure to repeating thoughts of doing poorly on a test and not getting into college, she might predict that she will stay anxious or grow even more anxious throughout the exposure. If, after repeating her worry thought for 20 minutes, Kara has become bored of the thought and her anxiety has decreased, she has one piece of evidence suggesting that fear does not build and build but, to the contrary, diminishes if she sits with her worries and doesn't try to avoid them.

Lastly, before starting an exposure, have your child rate how nervous they are that their fear will come true. At our clinic, we typically use a scale of 0 to 10 where 0 is not nervous at all and 10 is the most nervous possible—as good as terrified. We generally let kids provide whatever rating they feel is accurate. It's not an exact science, so if your child always starts at a 10, that's fine, but probably less helpful than if sometimes anxiety starts at a 7, at other times a 5, and occasionally a 9. Noticing that some situations are easier than others and that the initial anxiety decreases with practice can boost your child's confidence for more challenging exposures.

To give you an example of how rating works, while Michael and his mother are setting up the exposures, before putting their shoes on to cross the street and knock on the neighbor's door, his mom asks him how nervous he's feeling that the dog will bite him. She reminds him that 0 means *I'm not nervous at all the dog will bite me* and 10 means *I'm really terrified the dog will bite me.* Since being in his neighbor's house will be the closest Michael has ever been to this dog but knowing that he won't have to actually pet the dog, he replies that his nervousness is running at a 7. He and his mother are now ready to start his exposure.

## STEP 4: DOING AN EXPOSURE

After all the learning and preparation, it's time to do an exposure. Michael is at his neighbor's house, peering through the living room door at his neighbor sitting on the couch holding the dog on a leash. Michael's mother is by his side, trying to remember how to be a good exposure coach. The main things that Michael and his mother need to do are pay attention and stay positive.

## Pay attention

As we know, exposures are experiments to learn that the expectations that make safe situations scary are wrong and create space for new learning that these situations are reasonably safe. To learn something new, your child needs to pay attention to what is happening. And to support them, you as the parent need to pay attention to what your child is doing as well as what is happening during the exposure. The way we keep all parties focused is by repeatedly having your child rate how nervous they feel during an exposure.

***What to ask*** There are a few different ways to phrase the question about your child's current anxiety level. The most accurate wording of the question that captures what we want your child to be focusing on is: *How nervous are you that your fear will come true if you keep doing this exposure?*

This question usefully covers both your child's expectation about how likely they think their fears are to come true and how they are feeling in the moment. Although thoughts and feelings are different, we find they are so closely related, especially for younger kids, that it is not worth overcomplicating things by asking two separate questions.

However, this question is a bit of a mouthful, so you can shorten it to: *How nervous are you to keep doing this?* This question still makes it clear you are focusing on how they feel about continuing to do the feared activity. It focuses only on what your child feels rather than also talking about what they expect to happen, but the two are closely related, so it's a fine trade-off to keep things a little more efficient.

This wording works well for Michael, who is standing near the dog continuously without breaks.

Some exposures have natural pauses. When Maria goes from clothing store to clothing store, asking sales assistants, *Excuse me, where are the sweatshirts?* her father will wait outside and check in between each store. In this case he might ask her: *How nervous are you to keep doing this?* Or it might feel more natural to him to instead say: *How nervous are you to do it again?* Or even: *How nervous are you to talk to the next sales assistant?*

The goal for the check-in is to gauge how nervous Maria is to talk to the next person, at the next clothing store, not how relieved she is to be done talking to the last person. If her father was to ask *How nervous are you now?* Maria might say she's at a 2 simply because she's relieved to be back outside with her dad, even though she continues to be terrified to talk to the next sales assistant.

If a child's feelings during an exposure are not anxiety but rather feeling grossed out by germs or bothered by things being out of order, parents can change the wording of their questions to match the child's experience, such as, *How gross does this feel now?* or *How upset are you to keep doing this?*

***When to ask*** Kids give the first anxiety rating while setting up the exposure. Parents should ask for the next rating immediately after the child starts the exposure. Sometimes when kids start an exposure their anxiety goes up, because it was more challenging than they thought. Other times, anxiety immediately drops because the anticipation was worse than the activity. Both are fine, and recording the change helps your child learn from their experience.

As your child continues with an exposure, you should continue to repeat the same question about their anxiety. The goal is to help them stay focused on what they're doing and paying attention to what is happening, both to whether anything bad has occurred and also to changes in their anxious feelings.

How frequently you ask your child for an update on how they feel is a bit of an art. The goal is to ask frequently enough to catch changes in anxiety as they are happening but not so often that the question interferes with doing the exposure itself and becomes annoying. With an exposure that involves doing one action over and over, like talking to sales assistants, you will probably ask for a rating after each attempt. With continuous exposures, like petting a dog or sitting with germs or repeating thoughts, you will probably start by asking every 30 to 60 seconds and adjust the frequency based on the rate at which your child's anxiety seems to change.

***How to respond*** After each anxiety rating, parents should respond in a way that supports their child's learning. Anxiety often goes up during an exposure. Michael's anxiety might jump from a 7 to an 8 when he sees how big the dog looks up close. Or anxiety might rise as an exposure builds momentum. Alex might not be too nervous right after his mother leaves him alone in a room, but as it continues and she hasn't come back yet, his worries may begin to take over. In either case, when your child's anxiety rating goes higher, you can say something along the lines of, *You're doing great, the fact you're feeling more anxious means this is a really good exposure.*

> When your child's anxiety rating goes higher, you can say something along the lines of, *You're doing great, the fact you're feeling more anxious means this is a really good exposure.*

Exposures need to make your child feel anxious. If your child feels really nervous about a situation, but things then turn out well, that's surprising to them and makes for a powerful exposure. Having anxiety go up shows your child they're working hard, they're making a big effort, they're pushing themselves. It may be uncomfortable, but it's not a bad thing, it's an indicator that they are doing a really good exposure.

Often kids' anxiety ratings are the same as the last one and the one before that. This is especially true toward the beginning of an exposure and happens for one simple reason: Learning to feel safe in a feared situation is a slow process. Exposures are not quick and exciting; they are slow and challenging and they take time. But remember, one of the goals of an exposure is for kids to learn that they can handle feeling nervous. So, anxiety staying at the same level is not a problem, it's part of the process. You can respond to your child by saying: *You're doing a great job handling your anxiety, keep with it.*

When your child's anxiety rating comes down, this is where things are starting to move in the right direction and we really want kids to be paying attention. Parents should say, *That's great, what's bringing it down?* The answer we want the child to arrive at is: *I'm facing my fears and nothing bad is happening.* It is as simple as that. Any rating that goes down during an exposure—even by a single digit—is a success. This is why we use a rating system; it provides real-time encouragement and evidence of progress.

When your child's anxiety rating comes down, this is where things are starting to move in the right direction and we really want kids to be paying attention. Parents should say, *That's great, what's bringing it down?* The answer we want the child to arrive at is: *I'm facing my fears and nothing bad is happening.*

After Michael has been watching the dog for a few minutes, his mother notices he looks a little more relaxed and so decides it is a good time to once again ask, *How nervous are you to keep doing this?* This time Michael replies, *I don't know, maybe I am at a 6.* In response his mother says, *That's great! What's bringing it down?* To which Michael, because he is only 10 years old, replies, *I don't know, the dog just keeps panting.* So, his mother helps him along by clarifying, *That's right! You're facing your fears and nothing bad is happening.*

***What to look for*** Throughout the exposure, especially when anxiety comes down, parents need to make sure their child is not avoiding or doing rituals. Kids learn from exposures by noticing that their anxiety is decreasing solely because the exposure exercise is not as dangerous or overwhelming as they expected. To learn this, your child can't do avoidance behaviors, rituals, or seek reassurance that they might later believe were the reason they survived the exposure. If Michael hides behind his mother, he might assume that he was only safe because his mother protected him. Or if he repeatedly asks if the dog is nice and his mother keeps reassuring him that of course the neighbors have a nice dog, he might assume that he only felt better because of his mom's reassurance. This also means you don't want your child doing anything to decrease his or her anxiety during exposures, so no relaxation techniques, mindfulness exercises, five senses awareness, deep breathing, or distraction. We don't want your child to believe they felt better because they are getting good at relaxing, we want them to learn that they felt better because the situation was not dangerous or overwhelming.

Part of being an exposure coach therefore is keeping an eye out for any avoidance or rituals. We know kids will slip into some avoidance during exposures and when it happens, try not to get upset. Instead, calmly point out what they are doing and ask them if they can stop the avoidance. Michael's mother might say: *Standing behind me is avoiding the dog; to be successful you need to stand next to me.* If it's too hard for them to resist, we might overlook it for now but make it clear that the next time we do this exposure, it will have to be done without this avoidance behavior.

### Stay positive

You may have noticed that no matter what happens to your child's anxiety—up, down, stays the same—your response involves some form of encouragement along the lines of: *That's great!*

We know exposure is hard work and exposure coaching is in part being your child's cheerleader, warmly telling them that they are doing great and that you are proud of them. Keep in mind that while being warm and encouraging you need to refrain from giving reassurance. If you say, *You're doing a great job, I am so proud of you,* that's good cheerleading. But saying, *You will be fine, there is nothing to worry about,* is giving reassurance and stops your child from learning they can handle the exposure independently without you reminding them it is safe.

It is equally important for kids to have a positive attitude. If kids go in with the attitude that exposure therapy is a dumb idea that will never work and they're really mad at their parents, then they're going to spend all of their time and energy fighting the exposure and learn nothing from the experience. On the other hand, kids can set themselves up for success by going into an exposure with an open mind. Yes, they can acknowledge that the therapy sounds hard and challenging and a little unusual, but they see how it might be helpful and so give it the benefit of the doubt.

---

All of which brings us to the point where the exposure is live. Michael is watching the dog. Maria is going store to store asking for sweatshirts. Kara is repeating thoughts of failing an assignment rather than perfecting her homework. Alex is alone in his bedroom. And their parents are checking in on progress, looking out for avoidance, and tuned in to the difference between encouragement and reassurance. Your next question is probably: How do I know when my child is done with an exposure?

## STEP 5: ENDING AN EXPOSURE

If the goal of an exposure is to learn that a feared situation is reasonably safe and manageable, then an exposure is complete when a child has achieved this new learning. More specifically, we need to keep at an individual exposure until your child can answer these two questions:

1. Did my fear come true?
2. What happened to my anxiety?

Let's take the first question. One goal of an exposure is for a child to learn through their own experience that their fears are unlikely to come true. For that to happen, kids need to continue with any given planned exposure until they realize that what they were afraid would happen, has not happened, and probably won't or never will. This doesn't mean they have conquered their anxiety and can now do all previously feared activities. It simply means that in this given, specific instance they now have a new belief that says their fear is unlikely to come true. Michael needs to stand outside the living room doorway until he can say: *Okay, I get it, that dog isn't going to run over here and bite me today, he is just going to sit there and pant.* Michael doesn't have to acknowledge that the neighbors' dog is safe to play with, just that the current exposure is safe.

To complicate things a bit, it's important to point out that sometimes our fears do come true. Let's say down the road when Michael does an exposure to playing fetch with a dog, he is scared the dog will jump on him. Well, that fear may certainly come true, because dogs like to play and might jump at the stick in his hand before he throws it. Another example is social exposures, in which we worry that there might be an awkward pause and we won't know what to say, or that someone might say no when we ask for something, or that someone might ignore us when we give a compliment. These sorts of uncomfortable social situations happen all the time, including during exposures. In these situations, the goal of an exposure is for your child to learn that yes, their fear did come true, but it wasn't that bad and they were able to handle it.

Now let's look at that second question: *What happened to my anxiety?* The other goal for an exposure is for your child to learn that they can handle anxiety independently until it goes away without avoiding or doing rituals. Typically, in everyday (non-exposure) situations, kids only feel better after they escape the situation or do a ritual. This keeps them believing that anxiety won't go away without avoidance. With this in mind, you want to keep doing an exposure until your child's anxiety comes down. Ideally, we would like you to stick with it until your child's anxiety goes down to zero or close to zero, because that is a very satisfying experience for everyone involved. However, often—especially early on or when doing more difficult exposures—an anxiety rating of zero is not realistic. We usually set a goal of sticking with an exposure until your child's anxiety goes down by at least half, so if it starts at 8, we need to keep at it until your child's anxiety is 4 or less. There is no magic in coming down by half, it is just a good sign that your child has stuck with it long enough to learn that it gets easier with practice.

We can't control how we feel, so kids can't and shouldn't try to make their anxiety go down. Sometimes anxiety stays high, especially during the first exposure to a challenging situation. Maybe the anxiety will eventually come down, but we can't stick with an exposure all night. So, if your child's anxiety stays high, but they can say they were able to handle their fear and worry during the activity, then that is still a very successful exposure.

For your child to answer both of our wrap-up questions, they will need to stick with each exposure long enough to learn that their fears are unlikely to come true and their anxiety is manageable. This means that all planned exposures need to be repetitive.

Doing something once or briefly is not enough for your child to learn that a situation is safer than their anxiety tells them. For some exposures, the repetition is pretty straightforward. Your child simply needs to keep petting the dog, touching the doorknob, or repeating the thought until they have learned something new. Other exposures, especially those for social anxiety, which require talking to different people, can be more challenging to make repetitive. Despite this, social exposures still need to be as repetitive as any other exposures. If you are working on starting conversations in public, it can be helpful to go to a mall with multiple stores so your child has many salesclerks to start a conversation with and repeat the exposure as many times as needed.

Since learning that something is safe requires feeling better *before* ending the exposure, it is best to avoid setting a specific endpoint to an exposure. Typically, exposures can take anywhere from 10 to 20 minutes, which is a good length of time for moderate exposures. When working on your own without a therapist, give yourself 30 to 40 minutes for a planned exposure so you have time to stick with it as needed. If your child's anxiety is still high after that time, you can wrap it up and discuss how this practice will make the next time easier. However, if you have time and your child is willing to stick with it, you don't have to stop. A very challenging exposure can take an hour or even longer. Don't preset a time limit or certain number of repetitions with your child because that sets them up to focus on when they can escape, rather than on learning that nothing bad is happening.

Before closing the book on a planned exposure, spend a few minutes talking with your child about how it went. Review the answers to both of the questions we've just covered and ask more broadly what your child learned during the exposure. You can then complete the exposure record to chart progress. Talking about their experience and what they observed helps kids solidify what they learned from an exposure.

If, at the end of an exposure, your child says: *My fear came true, it was bad and my anxiety was out of control,* it's time to regroup. Either you tried to do something too hard, didn't stick with it long enough, or tried something that would be too challenging for any kid to handle. We will talk more about troubleshooting in the next chapter.

From my experience, the best way to know an exposure has been successfully completed is when a child can turn to you and say, *That wasn't so bad, I think I can do it again.*

## STEP 6: RINSE AND REPEAT

The key to planned exposures is repetition. Not only during a single exposure, to give your child time to learn that their fear is unlikely to come true, but also through returning to the same exposure again to learn that it gets easier with practice. There is no set number of times you and your child have to repeat an exposure. Some of the easier activities from the beginning of a fear ladder might only need to be done once before you can cross them off as mastered. More challenging exposures might have to be repeated multiple times with slight variations and changes along the way. You don't have to go in the order of your fear ladder, and it is not necessary to master one exposure before moving on to a harder one. Life is often unstructured

> The key to planned exposures is repetition.

and unpredictable, and this can be reflected in exposure therapy too. You and your child can jump from one activity to another and then back to the first. What is required, though, is consistency. If you don't do exposures, they won't work. Planning, doing, and reviewing exposures takes time and can be hard to fit into an already busy family schedule. As a parent overseeing your child's exposures, you are in charge of making sure exposures get done.

## STEP 7: WORKING IN THE MOMENT

Planned exposures prepare your child to handle their fears and worries when they occur in daily life. Moving from the structure and support of planned exposures to independently handling anxiety in the moment requires practice. On-the-fly exposures are the bridge between planned exposures and being able to do things independently. Once you and your child have completed some planned exposures, you should start actively looking for opportunities to apply that new learning spontaneously in naturally occurring situations. The steps for setting up and learning from on-the-fly exposures are similar to those for planned exposures, with the difference being that they are less structured and usually don't involve repetition. However, the goals of having a learning experience to challenge anxiety-provoking expectations are the same. You and your child can briefly set up on-the-fly exposures together and then review how they went and what your child learned. Once Michael and his mother have successfully completed planned exposures of petting the neighbor's dog, a playdate at the local park is now an opportunity for an on-the-fly exposure. When they see a woman walking her dog, Michael's mother might say, *Michael, here's a great chance to do an exposure. How nervous are you to ask that lady if you can pet her dog?* After Michael pets the dog, his mother briefly wraps things up by asking, *How did it go? Did anything bad happen?* The goal of on-the-fly exposures is for your child to be ready to handle similar situations on their own when they occur in daily life.

---

Now that we have detailed steps for doing exposure therapy with your child, let's go over what a timeline for doing exposures might look like.

# 9

# A Timeline for Doing Exposure Therapy

The timeline we'll now look at is not a firm prescription but rather a set of general guidelines based on 20 years of experience with hundreds of families in our clinic. As part of it, we'll also discuss signs to look out for that suggest you are making progress, as well as tips for troubleshooting when things are not going as well as you had hoped. Finally, we'll discuss when to seek further help and other potential treatment options should this become necessary.

Families who come to our clinic attend an average of seven or eight appointments spread out over a few months and complete an average of 25 planned exposures. Some families end treatment earlier and some continue for a lot longer. During this time families work through four stages: learning and planning; doing planned exposures; adding in on-the-fly exposures; and mastery and moving on with life.

All families have different experiences and go through these steps at different speeds, so don't feel as if you need to adhere closely to the milestones set out below. Rather, the following timeline is intended to break things up into manageable tasks to make the journey less overwhelming. Also, I hope to make it clear that working on anxiety and OCD through exposures is not a quick process but one that you need to stick with for weeks or months. And, third, do take your time. If your child wants to get going and move up the fear ladder more quickly, that's great. But if they want to go slow, and you rush and push too hard, that can make the process more stressful than it needs to be.

## A SUGGESTED TIMELINE FOR EXPOSURE THERAPY

### Phase 1: Learning and planning

The first few weeks of our timeline are focused on settling in, getting you and your child on the same page, learning, and making a plan.

*Week 1* Treatment in our clinic begins with an assessment where we meet with a child and their parents to discuss the concerns that have brought them in. We usually end this assessment deciding collectively that anxiety is a problem that we need to treat. Based on that, I suggest that, after you as the parent have finished reading this book, your goal for the first week is simply to talk about anxiety or OCD with your child and whether it's a problem that needs to be worked on. No decisions or fear ladders need to be made immediately. It might be helpful to give your child some time to think it over or, if it's age-appropriate, let them look over this book. If they don't want to look over the book, you can give them an overview of what exposure therapy entails. For younger children, you might start by asking them how often and when they feel scared or nervous or worried. You might then say something like, *Sometimes feeling scared or nervous makes kids sad and stops them from playing or having fun. Does that happen to you sometimes? Do you think that is something we should work on together?*

*Week 2* Most families don't immediately start therapy the week after the assessment because they need to arrange their calendar and schedule appointments. Mirroring this, you don't need to finish the last page of this book and rush straight into doing exposures either. Your goal for the second week is to decide with your child whether what they are experiencing is best described as an anxiety disorder. You can draw on Chapters 1 and 2 to determine if they are more scared or worried than we would expect in a given situation and which of the common anxiety conditions is most similar to their experience. Use this conversation to choose which chapter from Part 3 will best guide your treatment plan. Then you can move to completing an avoidance cycle with your child that describes their anxiety or OCD.

*Week 3* The next step is to make a plan to do exposures. You can use Part 2 of this book to introduce your child to the mechanics of how exposures break the avoidance cycle, should they be curious and want more information about the treatment you are proposing. Then you can work together to build a fear ladder—several, if needed—using Chapter 8 and the examples from Part 3 for reference.

### Phase 2: Doing planned exposures

The next few weeks are then focused on learning how to do an exposure through your own hands-on practice, with a view to achieving initial small wins and confidence-building success.

*Week 4* Now it's time to launch the first exposure. This means starting easy with the goal of you and your child learning how to do exposures through an initial practice. You can then repeat that first introductory exposure and subsequent, fairly easy exposures at least three times during the week.

*Week 5* Now that you and your child are comfortable with setting up, doing, and learning from exposures, you can shift focus to building on success. During this week, aim to do at least three planned exposures, sticking with items toward the easier end of the fear ladder but beginning to slowly work your way up. Once again, if your child is ready to move ahead, don't hold them back. But also, don't feel any pressure to push your child too fast.

*Week 6* By now, I hope that you and your child are seeing progress and have been able to cross off some early items from the fear ladder as successfully mastered. During this week, you can build on previous successful exposures by stepping up from low-level exposures to moderate-level exposures. As before, aim to do at least three exposures this week and gradually make each one more challenging than its predecessor.

### Phase 3: Adding in on-the-fly exposures

As we now enter the second half of our treatment timeline, we are going to add in a new focus on applying what we have learned through planned exposures to daily life.

*Week 7* You and your child should continue to do a minimum of three planned exposures this week, all in the moderate range in terms of difficulty, and keep working your way up the fear ladder. To introduce the idea of doing on-the-fly exposures, pick an easier item from the fear ladder that your child has successfully completed planned exposures to, and work together to do related on-the-fly exposures during the flow of daily life.

*Week 8* By now, you are about two-thirds of the way through the treatment timeline. This is a good opportunity to review progress and begin focusing on what your child still needs to accomplish. I encourage families to cross off all the items on the fear ladder that their child has already mastered as a clear marker of progress. Then, based on your success so far, start refining what you and your child think would be the ultimate, most challenging exposure to demonstrate that your child has mastered their anxiety or OCD. With that goal in mind, sketch out a plan for how you are going to complete the remaining exposures over the next month. And of course, continue to do at least three planned exposures this week for items sitting at the more challenging end of the fear ladder. You can also now bring in two more on-the-fly-exposures, so the new learning permeates your child's everyday schedule.

*Week 9* Exposures should now be solidly toward the high end of the fear ladder. Your efforts can be divided between ensuring your child completed a couple of planned exposures to challenging items as well as a couple of on-the-fly exposures to activities that used to be in the moderate range but are now on their way to being mastered.

## Phase 4: Mastery and moving on

During the final weeks we want to help your child demonstrate mastery of anxiety or OCD and also address any remaining fears you might have missed, so your child can move on with their life, no longer incapacitated by anxiety or OCD.

*Week 10* This week is all about finishing off exposures near the top of the fear ladder in preparation for next week's mastery exposure. In addition, you can respond in the moment to any daily situations that cause anxiety for your child by bringing out on-the-fly exposures, when it's appropriate.

***Week 11*** This is the week you and your child have been building up to over the past couple of months: the mastery exposure. This week your child will complete the challenging exposure that you and your child have designed to address their biggest fear, an activity that is more challenging than what would actually happen in daily life. The mastery exposure needs to be something so awesome that it inspires your child to say once they're done: *Because I did that exposure during therapy, I now know I can do anything!* In addition to completing the mastery exposure, you can supplement your child's exposure regimen by continuing to do regular on-the-fly exposures.

***Week 12*** With the mastery exposure out of the way and most items crossed off the fear ladder, it's time to begin wrapping up the active phase of treatment. While our focus is mostly on handling anxiety and OCD in the moment through on-the-fly exposures, you can finish off any lingering planned exposures for items that might have slipped through the cracks up until now. And prepare for less structure as you and your child move on with life. From your experience over the past couple of months, you and your child hopefully feel comfortable with exposure. Even though your active focus on treating anxiety or OCD is ending, facing fears rather than avoiding and doing rituals is a mindset that you and your child will need to continue. Take some time to review and celebrate what you have accomplished and what activities in life your child is now back to enjoying. At the same time, prepare a corner of your mind for the probability that anxiety is likely to come back. If that does happen, you can simply

> Keep in mind this timeline is set out to give you a suggested structure and pacing. It is okay to take longer or go faster based on your child's needs and the rest of life's demands.

dust off this book, make a new plan, draw up a new fear ladder, complete a run of exposures, and get your child once again back on track.

Keep in mind this timeline is set out to give you a suggested structure and pacing. It is okay to take longer or go faster based on your child's needs and the rest of life's demands.

With this road map for treatment in place, let's now focus on what to look for to make sure you are progressing and are prepared to respond to potential problems that you might encounter along the way.

## HOW DO I KNOW WHEN EXPOSURE THERAPY IS WORKING?

As you work through the timeline, you will at some point wonder if you are on the right track. An early sign of success is when a child starts participating actively in the planning process. They may readily share their fears and worries as you complete the avoidance cycle or generate ideas for the fear ladders. These are good signs, but enthusiasm at this stage is neither required nor expected. So don't be disheartened if your child is quiet or reluctant to participate in planning exposures and making a fear ladder.

Once exposures are underway, you'll begin to see signs of success during planned exposures. Initially we are not expecting quick changes in daily anxiety or your child's ability to handle real-world feared situations. Rather, therapy is on track when designated exposures go well. If after a child finishes an exposure you can already see that they're calmer, less nervous, and proud of their accomplishment, at least for the moment, then this is an early sign you're on the right track. One rewarding aspect of exposure therapy is that if a child's anxiety goes down during an exposure, over five, ten, twenty minutes, that's immediate feedback things are getting better.

Another marker of success is when an exposure is easier the next time your child completes it. I find this to be one of the most satisfying experiences, when a child who previously struggled to manage anxiety through an exposure the first time around completes the second round feeling calmer and more confident. The next milestone of progress is working up the fear ladder. If your child is moving from easier to more challenging exposure, this suggests you are on the right track. When a child and their parent agree that planned exposures to an item are no longer needed, I encourage them to check that item off the fear ladder as mastered.

The final measure of progress, and the one we are most eager to see, is when your child starts doing activities they previously avoided. This might be Michael petting his aunt's dog during a visit, or Maria staying late to chat with the other girls after skating, or Alex's mother realizing she has not had to check on him after bedtime all week. Change often occurs gradually and little improvements can slip by unnoticed. Be on the lookout for chances to celebrate small victories and discrete moments of success.

## TROUBLESHOOTING

Facing one's fears is challenging, and it's very normal for exposure therapy to be difficult. Coaching your child through exposures is often not very straightforward, and there are times when parents can feel uncertain about what they're supposed to be doing and have a lot of questions about how to make things more successful.

With this in mind, here are some of the more common challenges families encounter during exposure therapy, so you can have an eye out for pitfalls and obstacles that might crop up.

### I don't know what I am supposed to do

Most parents are not experts in mental health, and therefore it takes time to learn about anxiety disorders and other emotional problems that may be impacting their child. On top of that, helping your child do exposure therapy involves learning a new skill, and this takes time and practice. Give yourself space and permission to learn; you don't have to understand everything or get it right from day one. As long as you are working with your child and taking small steps, just get started and work things out together as you go. Mistakes are opportunities to learn. We often learn better by watching someone else demonstrate something first and getting hands-on support after that. If you are not feeling confident enough to get started on your own, no problem, you are now a very knowledgeable consumer about what you need from a mental health professional. A couple of sessions with a therapist specializing in exposure therapy might be enough to get you going until you're ready to carry on at home.

### Is this the right approach for my child?

Working on anxiety involves continuing to gather information and assess the situation from one step to the next. Sometimes when families come to see us for concerns about anxiety, by the end of the assessment we decide that their concerns don't fit how we understand anxiety disorders. Occasionally, what seems like an anxiety disorder the first time we meet starts to look like something else as we begin treatment. Sometimes a child's symptoms don't fit well into the avoidance cycle or don't match up with any of the anxiety diagnoses, and we decide their symptoms are better described as something else, like depression, adjustment to stress, or behavior problems. Sometimes we can't find anything to put on a fear ladder and that leads us to change our understanding of the child's symptoms. If building a fear ladder or doing exposures doesn't seem like the right fit, either practically or instinctively, then you can go back over this book and reevaluate again whether an anxiety disorder is the best description for the concerns you have for your child. It may also be a good time to seek a professional evaluation to identify the right path for your child.

### Exposures don't make my child nervous

There are several reasons why exposures may not make your child nervous. If this is happening early on, it might simply be because the exposures are too easy and, if that's the case, then you just need to increase the challenge. Other times, kids might be expressing reluctance to do something uncomfortable. They might say something like, *I'm not nervous to talk to other people, I just don't want to do it.* But if despite what they're saying, they look nervous to you, carry on with exposures.

For some sets of symptoms, it may be harder to bring on anxiety during planned exposures. For example, a child with social anxiety who only struggles with peers they are familiar with and will see again, such as classmates at school, may not feel nervous practicing social interactions with salesclerks at the mall. Similarly, some children with just-right OCD symptoms feel they have to tap or repeat things until it feels just right, but this sensation doesn't happen when we try to purposely bring it on during planned exposures. In both these and similar situations, planned exposures are still good opportunities to learn how to do exposures. It's like soccer practice: dribbling and passing drills are not the same as a game, but if you do these drills consistently you will have better ball control come game time. It's the same with exposures. Even if planned exposures don't cause anxiety, the more often your child goes through the steps of doing an exposure, the more likely your child will be successful taking these steps during on-the-fly exposures when social anxiety or just-right OCD symptoms come on spontaneously.

In some cases, planned exposures don't bring on anxiety because we have missed the mark. As we discussed above, it may be a sign that an anxiety disorder is not the best description for what your child is experiencing. In which case, return to the descriptions of anxiety, the avoidance cycle, and the descriptions of other mental health conditions to make sure you have accurately understood your child's experience.

Other times, a child may have an anxiety disorder, but we haven't yet nailed down what sets off their fears and worries. For example, we might at first decide a child is experiencing separation anxiety because he is really nervous and clinging to his parents before going to school. But when we start treatment, he breezes through the exposures, apparently having no problem at all sitting in a room alone, staying home while parents run errands, or going to a friend's house alone. At the same time, he continues to be extremely nervous before school. When we take another look at his avoidance cycle, we realize he is nervous about going to school because his teacher started doing show and tell and assigning kids to work with classmates they don't mix with often. Based on this, we refocus the fear ladder to social anxiety and start doing social anxiety exposures and soon enough find out that we are now on the right course of treatment.

### My child is refusing to cooperate with exposures

Exposures are challenging, and sometimes kids are not eager to cooperate. This is when we go back to our motivation plan of taking small steps, using attention through praise and ignoring, setting goals and rewards, and drawing up consequences. However, if this is not enough or your child is not only resisting exposures but is also generally argumentative and acting out, such as by refusing to stop playing video games, clean up their toys, or come to dinner, then we recommend pausing exposures for anxiety and switching focus instead to improving cooperation through behavior management.

### Exposures make my child too anxious

Parents are sometimes concerned about whether their child can handle the anxiety that comes with exposure or if being too nervous during exposures will make their child's anxiety worse. With this, there are a couple of things to keep in mind. First, there is nothing wrong with kids feeling nervous, even very nervous. Learning that they can push through and handle those feelings independently is a very empowering experience. However, it is normal for parents to be uncomfortable and anxious and thoroughly dislike seeing their child being anxious and upset and not being allowed to do anything to soothe them. It can be helpful for parents to prepare for this ahead of time, because when parents don't think exposure is right for their child, kids may sense that and feel more anxious and uncertain themselves.

Kids can sometimes feel overwhelmed by high anxiety during exposures because they are moving too quickly up the fear ladder. This can result from overenthusiastic parents pushing the process too hard (and I say this with no judgment, because when our children are not feeling well, we want to see them get better as fast as possible) or from kids wanting to work hard or impress their parents and not realizing how difficult an exposure would actually be. In either situation, the solution is to take a step back and slow down or add some smaller steps to the fear ladder.

With all this in mind, a child cannot avoid feeling nervous during an exposure because that is fundamental to the process. If your child experiences big emotions even with the smallest steps, then you can calmly and warmly wait out their anxiety in the moment. As with most challenges to exposure therapy, if you consistently do not feel comfortable with the amount of anxiety your child is experiencing, then it might be the time to seek professional support.

### My child's anxiety is not coming down during exposures

Parents understandably worry if it seems their child's anxiety is not coming down during exposures. The first thing to consider is whether you and your child are giving the exposure enough time. Exposures usually take around 20 minutes—at least that's the typical time we spend doing them in our treatment groups at the clinic. But on occasion, exposures might take 30 or 40 minutes or even an hour before a child's anxiety decreases, and while that's a long time, it's the sign of a valuable and challenging exposure. Practically speaking, we don't expect you and your child to stick with most exposures for more than 40 minutes or so, simply because you have other daily responsibilities to manage.

When families first get started, even two minutes of their child sitting very upset and anxious and stressed can seem like a very long time to both parents and the child. As is often the recommendation for common barriers experienced during exposure, start small and build confidence in the process with easier activities that are unlikely to take a long time to master.

In some cases, anxiety does not decrease *during* an exposure, but it does decrease *between* exposures, and that's fine. We can't control anxiety, but we can learn to handle and manage it. If anxiety stays high during an exposure, you can say to your child, *That's perfectly normal, you learned that you can handle feeling nervous, and it will probably be easier the next time.* That's a successful exposure and there is no need for concern whatsoever. And if indeed your child is less nervous the next time you try that exposure, you are on the right track.

Sometimes, anxiety stays high when kids are worrying about a different fear than the one you are working on at the moment. Let's say Kara is working on repeating her worry thought about getting poor grades and failing to get into college. While she is doing that, her thoughts drift to fears of failing the math test she has later in the week. In this moment we are focusing an exposure on her college worries, because that fear was the first item on her fear ladder. In this situation, Kara tries to separate her anxiety. She keeps track of her fear about college, which we expect to decrease with repetition during the exposures, even though her more immediate worries stay high. Through this exposure Kara learns to handle worries about the future, and we can use that confidence to handle more immediate worries, like the upcoming test, in later exposures.

Some kids may get stuck and need some help from a parent to achieve a successful exposure. Kids may realize that if their anxiety comes down, that means they will then have to move up to a more challenging exposure and with that, get closer to being more independent in daily life. Anxiety about moving forward keeps them reporting continued high anxiety, even when they outwardly look calm. Other kids may have trouble using the number scale to rate their anxiety, especially younger kids who may find using numbers to track feelings too abstract. In both cases, parents can praise their child's success in handling an exposure and then use their judgment as a parent about when to move on to the next step.

### Exposures are not helping in daily life

If anxiety is not coming down from one exposure to another or success is not transferring from planned exposures to real daily situations, make sure nothing is interfering with your child's learning. If kids are distracting themselves, doing rituals, or relying on parents for reassurance during planned exposures, their anxiety may decrease in the moment, but they aren't prepared to handle the situations in real life on their own.

If you and your child are successfully getting rid of avoidance during exposures, make sure you are repeating each exposure enough times for your child to realize their fears are unlikely to come true. Being repetitive also means doing the same exposure multiple times on different days, in different places, before your child is ready to handle the situation spontaneously in everyday life.

Sometimes avoidance and rituals become a habit that continues even after anxiety and OCD have improved. It is often necessary for parents to make an active effort through implementing the motivation plan to encourage kids to apply what they have learned during planned exposures to spontaneous daily situations.

## SEEKING HELP

I hope that you can take the information in this book, run with it, and not need additional help. But for many families a more realistic goal may be that the knowledge you have gained helps you ensure that your child receives the right treatment.

If you want to find mental health care for your child, the quickest route is often to see your family doctor or pediatrician for advice. They may be able to help connect you with a local therapist. Schools can also be an easily accessible resource, and many have counselors or therapists practicing in the school building.

Unfortunately, it can be difficult to find a therapist close to you with expertise in using exposure for anxiety disorders or OCD. Professional organizations like the Association for Behavioral and Cognitive Therapies (www.abct.org), the Anxiety and Depression Association of America (www.adaa.org), and the International OCD Foundation (www.iocdf.org) offer excellent resources and allow you to search for therapists that specialize in anxiety or OCD in your area. There are also intensive treatment programs, such as ours at Mayo Clinic, that are designed for families that don't have access to exposure therapy in their home area.

As a parent you are going to have to be prepared to advocate for your child when navigating the mental health system, and this is where this book can come in helpful. You now have a guide and road map to understand anxiety disorders and OCD and how to treat them with exposure therapy as well as be an informed consumer when searching for the right therapist.

It may take considerable effort to find a suitable therapist who offers exposure therapy. More often you will likely find therapists who offer cognitive behavioral therapy (CBT). CBT includes exposures and has a lot of research showing its effectiveness but also adds in other strategies. Working with a therapist who offers high-caliber CBT will likely be helpful should a professional focusing on exposure therapy not be available.

Besides CBT, other treatment options you may encounter involve working with therapists who only use coping strategies or mindfulness or spend sessions talking and being supportive. This type of treatment can be comforting and helpful for other problems and issues but is not as targeted at solving the unique problems at the heart of anxiety disorders.

If you find a therapist you like, they may be willing to help you work through the exposures outlined in this book, even if they don't specialize in anxiety disorders or OCD. That might give you professional support to feel more confident getting started.

Medication is another option and often the first one offered to families. The approach in our clinic is to begin with exposure therapy and see how much progress we can make. If kids start therapy and medication at the same time and get better, you don't know which one was helpful and should be continued and which one can be stopped. Kids frequently improve enough with exposure therapy that they don't need other treatment.

## MOVING ON

Whether you tackle exposure therapy on your own or work with a therapist, at some point you and your child are going to want to be done and move on with your lives. When it comes to treating childhood anxiety disorders with exposure, we have two main treatment goals:

1. Help kids feel better—less scared, nervous, and worried
2. Help kids do all the things they want to do and need to do to be successful

These goals are subjective, and there's no clear-cut answer as to when you have achieved either one sufficiently. To help answer these questions we can look back to where we started. What were the concerns that led you to seek help, and have they improved? Therapy should be very problem-focused. Take the things that are getting in the way of your child living their best life and work methodically on them until your concerns have improved.

It can also help to review the three jobs kids have that we touched on earlier. Is anxiety or OCD still interfering with your child's ability to participate in school, do fun activities with friends, or take part in family activities? Improvements in functioning are important because we can never really know how our child, or anybody else for that matter, feels. We can only judge what we see in terms of how people act and behave. So, you want to set your goals on actions and activities that can be objectively measured.

We do, however, want our children to feel better. If we look back at our definition of an anxiety disorder, it involves *problems resulting from consistently feeling more nervous, worried, or scared in a situation than would be expected.* So, one end goal is for your child to be calmer, more confident, and less worried and nervous. However, this does not mean that they are never anxious, or even overly anxious at times. Anxiety, fear, worry, and nervousness are normal experiences that we all have, and some people will always tend to feel that way more than others. Some people are calmer, some are more anxious.

Success with exposure therapy does not mean arriving at the absence of anxiety, but rather your child feeling less nervous and able to do what they need and want to do despite feelings of anxiety.

Looking farther down the road, no matter how successful we are at reducing anxiety and OCD, we need to expect that fears and worries, obsessions and compulsions are likely to return. We know it is likely to happen, but the good news is that just because these symptoms return does not mean they are going to be as severe or problematic as they were before. You and your child now have the tools to face fear and get back on track.

Anxiety is not something you work on and then it's done. It's more like exercising, eating well, and getting good sleep—all the things we have to continuously try to do to stay healthy. Facing one's fears rather than avoiding them becomes a way of life.

The end goal is for your child to be able to live their best life and for you as a family to be able to do the things you need and want to do. Please do remember, should the current treatment you're following end up not being sufficient, there are always higher levels of care and support.

## PART 2 CONCLUSION

This brings us to the end of what we set out to learn about exposure therapy. Hopefully you feel confident that exposure is the best treatment for your child's anxiety, and with that, you are poised to attempt exposure therapy together. We're now ready to move into Part 3 of this book, where we will delve into the specifics of how to apply what you learned about exposure therapy to each of the most common forms of anxiety and OCD.

# PART 3

# Applying Exposure Therapy to the Most Common Anxiety Disorders

In this part, we're going to bring everything we've learned so far about anxiety disorders and exposure therapy together and apply it to each of the most common anxiety disorders as well as OCD. You'll learn how to plan and carry out exposures for each condition, what to do with problems or issues that may arise during the process, and what signs of success to look for. You don't need to read straight through or linger on chapters that don't apply; instead, go straight to chapters on the conditions that you believe best fit your child's fears and worries and get to work.

# 10

# Exposure Therapy for Social Anxiety Disorder

Social anxiety is when a child feels overly nervous or worried when talking to or being around other people, especially other kids their age. This fear and anxiety can occur in any situation in which kids worry they might be judged by others. Social anxiety disorder differs from typical shyness in terms of intensity and the problems it causes. The anxiety crosses the line and becomes a problem when fears of being judged by others prevent children from doing the things they want or need to do.

When deciding if your child's experience is consistent with social anxiety disorder, it is important to explore whether there are other explanations for their fear and worry. For instance, if your child is being bullied or teased at school, their dread and fear of social situations is an understandable response to that situational stress, and the best plan would be to help put a stop to the bullying or find a way for your child to avoid or more effectively deal with the peers who are mistreating them. Similarly, if your child is pretty outgoing but has trouble making or keeping friends, their worry and distress about relationships may accurately reflect difficulty with interpersonal skills, in which case you will want to focus on helping them develop and improve their ability to relate to their peers.

If you decide that excessive fear and worry about judgment in social situations is the problem, whether your child gets very anxious about talking in class, ordering food at a restaurant, participating in sports or games, or meeting new people, the exercises in this chapter may be helpful.

## STEP 1: BUILDING FROM THE SOCIAL ANXIETY AVOIDANCE CYCLE

A successful exposure plan needs to be individually tailored to your child's needs using the avoidance cycle.

### What sets off social anxiety?

First, we need to identify what sets off your child's anxiety. Social anxiety is typically set off by things in the world around us, most often situations in which kids need to talk to their peers or other people or when they may be observed by others. There are many different types of social situations and not all will give your child feelings of anxiety.

Some children get more nervous in performance situations—reading aloud in class, acting in a school play, singing in a school musical, answering a question in class, competing in a basketball game, playing in a school concert, or giving a presentation in class. Others might get more nervous in unstructured social situations, like initiating conversations, meeting other kids at the start of a new school year, joining a club, finding people to sit with during lunch, or making small talk in the hallways between classes. And then there are kids whose anxiety is set off by talking to adults, especially in public situations such as the school principal, a teacher, or a sports coach.

These children may also be nervous to order food at restaurants, ask questions of store clerks, or check out with you at the grocery store. Sometimes children feel nervous simply being in public where people may be watching and observing them. For many kids with social anxiety, all of the above situations may set off their fears and worries.

In addition to situations and activities, for some kids social anxiety is set off by memories of awkward social situations or physical feelings of anxiety or embarrassment, like blushing or sweating, which lead to the same withdrawal and avoidance as social anxiety that relates to real-time, everyday scenarios.

## Expectations that make social situations scary

Once you've identified the situations that set off your child's anxiety, the next thing to do is pinpoint the expectations that cause your child to feel nervous in these situations when most of their peers enjoy them or feel only somewhat uncomfortable. As we have learned, there are two main expectations that drive fear and worry—*something bad will happen* and *I won't be able to handle this*—both apply to kids with social anxiety.

A core component of social anxiety is the fear of being judged negatively. However, the type of feared judgment often differs based on the situation in which kids feel anxious. Kids who get nervous speaking in performance situations may have expectations that they will make mistakes, perform poorly, and be judged as not good enough, smart enough, or talented enough. Kids who are more nervous about talking to peers may be more afraid that they will do something embarrassing and everyone will think they're uncool or unlikable. And when kids are nervous around authority figures they are typically concerned about getting in trouble, being a burden, or irritating others. For many children with social anxiety, expectations can occur in any combination of the above.

Despite the importance of expecting negative judgment in social anxiety, it's important to note that some kids don't describe these specific worries. Younger kids especially are more likely to simply say that talking to others is scary and they don't know why. Teens may add that they know it's unlikely that people will laugh at them or be mean but that they still feel nervous. If this is the case, you might describe the child's expectation as believing they can't handle talking to people or they have to avoid being around people to feel okay.

### Avoidance of social situations

Next, we need to identify what avoidance strategies your child uses to stay away from the situations they fear and in doing so, miss out on the opportunity to learn that these situations are not as bad as they expect them to be.

The most common form of avoidance for kids with social anxiety disorder is partial physical avoidance, which is when kids can't completely avoid a situation but try to avoid as much of it as possible when they are in the midst of it. For example, these kids can't avoid going to class, but when in class, they are careful never to raise their hand to answer a question asked by a teacher. Or because of anxiety around playing on the school football team, a teen might arrive at practice at the last minute and rush home quickly afterward to avoid the banter and socializing among teammates in the locker room.

Partial avoidance due to social anxiety can also include a child keeping their head down while walking in the hallways between classes at school, avoiding eye contact to make sure no one talks to them, or purposefully reading a book before class to put up a wall against being greeted by fellow classmates.

As many parents of socially anxious children know, full avoidance of anxiety-provoking activities can also occur. Complete avoidance involves not signing up for sports, clubs, and other extracurricular activities. Or not attending school dances or sporting events. Or eating lunch in the library. It may grow to include staying home from school on days there is a presentation due or even transitioning to online school or homeschooling.

Kids with social anxiety often rely on others to help avoid feared social interactions. As we saw earlier, parents may be asked to order food in restaurants or communicate with teachers. A more subtle form of avoidance that is easy to overlook is when kids rehearse what they are going to say over and over again, essentially overpreparing, to minimize the chance of making a mistake or being judged. For example, a teenager might repeat, *I'll have the cheeseburger with fries,* over and over, before the waitress comes to her family's table to ask for their order.

---

Let's go back to 16-year-old Maria, our overly shy figure skater. She's going to guide us through applying what we have learned to social anxiety. To remind you of her story, Maria was struggling to meet new friends at school, give presentations, and hang out with other girls before skating practice. When Maria and her parents mapped out her avoidance cycle, they found that situations that most frequently set off her anxiety involved talking to other kids her age. What she feared most was doing something foolish that would lead her peers to laugh at her and, as a result, see no value in being friends with her. Although she outright avoided some school activities and relied on her parents to order for her at restaurants, most of her avoidance strategies involved finding ways to dodge direct conversation when at school or during activities by looking busy, avoiding eye contact, or leaving early.

## STEP 2: BUILDING SOCIAL ANXIETY FEAR LADDERS

Now that we've used the avoidance cycle to organize Maria's social anxiety, let's use that cycle to build a fear ladder. As we learned earlier, fear ladders are treatment plans in the form of lists of exposure activities that can be done to face the feared situations that set off your child's anxiety. Since social anxiety is most often set off by situations and activities, most exposures on a fear ladder for social anxiety will be action exposures. Start off making a fear ladder by listing all the core social situations that set off your child's social anxiety from the avoidance cycle and then expand upon it. Make sure to add all the activities and situations that make your child nervous or that they avoid. For Maria this list might look like this: talking to kids in class at lunch, skating practice, ordering food, shopping, making plans with friends, meeting new people, presentations, and asking for help.

The next step is to turn the listed feared situations into exposures by breaking down challenging items into smaller steps that can be practiced at a set time to test expectations that something bad will happen. With social anxiety, the early steps on a fear ladder are normal activities, like asking questions in public or giving a presentation to parents. Through these early exposures, kids learn they generally do a fine job and they are unlikely to make big mistakes that lead to people laughing at them and judging them.

These types of exposures are a great first step but may leave your child worrying about what would happen if they did make a mistake, such as saying something embarrassing. This is particularly important for social anxiety because in any given social interaction, there is a good chance of making a mistake, being judged, stumbling over our words, or having an awkward pause.

In order to learn that life carries on even when we do something embarrassing, the later, more challenging activities on a fear ladder should involve purposely making mistakes, something we call social mishap exposures. In Maria's case, social mishap exposures might involve purposely and deliberately stumbling over her words when talking to a salesclerk in a store or ordering an item that is not on the menu, such a pizza at an ice cream shop.

The truth is, people often don't react or care as much as we thought they would when we make mistakes, but we can only learn that through our own experience. Social mishap exposures that engineer your child's worst-case scenarios are often the ultimate mastery exposure. However, it's important not to get carried away. The goal is not to humiliate your child or do something that leads to negative attention from their peers. Social mishaps should mimic common mistakes or be carried out in appropriate settings away from your child's peer groups and therefore be unlikely to impact negatively on your child's reputation.

When organizing our lists of potential exposures into fear ladders, we have found that it can be helpful for children with social anxiety to make three separate ladders. We often start with a fear ladder focused on talking in public situations. These activities are some of the more feasible to set up and allow for direct practice. Maria might begin with walking in public and making eye contact with people and simply saying *Hi.* Or she might ask single questions of people in public, starting with asking a store clerk a question like: *Where can I find scarves, please?* Staff working in a customer-facing job will often be easier to approach because they are a captive audience and generally, by profession, tend to be friendly. You can make these exposures more challenging by extending the interaction with multiple questions. Maria could still start by asking where the scarves are, but then add, *How are you today?* or *Which scarf do you like best?* In a restaurant, she could ask what the soup of the day is, then ask what flavors of ice cream are available.

You can also add social mishap exposures to the ladder and have your child do things like deliberately drop coins or textbooks in the mall in order to draw attention in an embarrassing way. Ultimate mastery exposures in public settings often involve making a mistake and having to be assertive. Maria could go up to a counter to purchase an item and then explain that she forgot her purse or, alternatively, take an item to a changing room and bring it out and ask the clerk if they have it in a different size.

Here is an example of what a fear ladder to talking in public places often looks like. You might find this ladder works as it is for your child, or it can be a start for tailoring to better match your child's specific fears.

### Talking in public places

1. Call a store and ask what time they close or for directions
2. Ask expected questions in public (e.g., to clerks about store items or for directions at an information desk)
3. Order food at restaurants
4. Ask people in public for directions to someplace that is obvious (such as the building you're standing in front of)
5. Call stores and make mistakes while talking (say the wrong word, use a long pause)
6. Politely compliment a stranger in a safe setting (e.g., *I like your coat*)
7. Ask questions about the menu before ordering food
8. Start conversations, more than an expected question, with store clerks (e.g., talk about a gift you are looking for)
9. Ask unexpected questions in public (e.g., ask people who are walking for the time or directions)
10. Change your order
11. Pay for items at stores on your own
12. Check out with a store cashier and apologize for not having enough money to pay for the item
13. Make mistakes while asking questions in public (e.g., try ordering pizza in an ice cream shop)

Given the frequency with which social anxiety centers around other kids and the importance of making friends, we often build a second fear ladder for interacting with peers. This will likely be the most important fear ladder in Maria's treatment. Exposures in this category can include sending texts or making phone calls to friends and acquaintances, making plans, going to the park with peers, or going out to find kids of a similar age to say hello to. Other useful exposures can include saying *Hi* to a kid your child doesn't usually say hello to at school, starting a conversation with someone different every day at school, or sitting with peers at lunchtime and suggesting a topic for conversation. One of the challenges of doing these exposures is that parents can't always be around to keep an eye on progress, such as with exposures that happen during the school day. However, parents may be able to more directly observe their kids' social exposures at other times, such as before or after extracurricular activities. In addition, some of the activities from the public interaction fear ladder can help with this ladder's items too, such as starting conversations with younger, similar-aged salesclerks.

The following fear ladder can help you work on your child's fears about interacting with other kids. Initial, easier items can include role-playing or short interactions with more familiar peers. Mastery exposures can involve exposures in real-world settings, like going to a school dance or making mistakes while talking to peers. Social mishaps with peer interactions are usually subtle, such as a long pause or misspeaking, things that happen all the time but still directly challenge the anxiety-causing expectations that making mistakes will lead to a horrible outcome.

### Interacting with peers

1. Practice having a conversation with someone you know, like a therapist or family member

2. Make eye contact and say "Hi" to people while out in public
3. Give a compliment to someone
4. Ask other kids a question
5. Start conversations with someone your age you don't know well
6. Join conversations that others are having
7. Suggest an idea for social plans (e.g., which restaurant or movie to go to)
8. Disagree with something a friend says
9. Purposely make mistakes during a conversation (e.g., a long pause or misspeak)
10. Contact classmates and ask about homework
11. Call or message friends you haven't talked to for a while
12. Make plans to get together with a friend
13. Join a club or organization
14. Attend social events and talk to people

Since children spend a lot of their time at school, it is perhaps not surprising that the third fear ladder we draw up often focuses on social anxiety around speaking in class. Exposures in this category can start off with an action such as your child giving presentations to you at home, then move up to practicing the same with a small group of extended family or family friends. Or it could look like setting a goal for your child to raise their hand in one class per day and ask a question and then arranging with their teacher in advance that they will send an email home to you confirming that your child carried out the exposure. Mastery exposures for this fear ladder could involve giving presentations with intentional mistakes or without time to prepare. Here is a typical fear ladder for classroom-related exposures that you can use as is or adapt more precisely to your child's fears.

Talking in class

1. Read a presentation in front of someone you know (e.g., a therapist or family member)
2. Give presentations without preparation in front of someone you know (e.g., a therapist or family member)
3. Give presentations in front of a small group
4. Practice answering or asking questions in a group setting, like a therapy group or club
5. Practice answering a question wrong or asking an obvious question in a group setting, like a therapy group or club
6. Answer or ask questions in a class
7. Give a presentation to your teacher
8. Give a presentation to your teacher and a few classmates
9. Purposely make mistakes—a long awkward pause, mispronounce a word—while giving a presentation
10. Give presentations in class

---

These three unique fear ladders, with additions and revisions, frequently form the basis for social anxiety treatment plans at our clinic. However, you don't have to follow this three-ladder approach if it doesn't fit your child's fears. Remember that exposure therapy needs to be tailored, appropriate, and accurate to your child's fears.

In addition to the action-oriented exposures listed so far, it can be helpful to add thought exposures to anxiety-producing memories about previous social situations. However, we generally don't do imaginal exposures in which a child pictures a social situation in their mind, like presenting in class, as this will be less effective than an action exposure. If your child is having trouble getting started, we generally break action exposures down into smaller steps, like role-playing with a parent, rather than turning to imaginal exposures.

## STEP 3: SETTING UP SOCIAL ANXIETY EXPOSURES

Once fear ladders are drawn up, you can move on to setting up planned exposures. As social anxiety exposures typically involve being in places with other people, setup and advance planning is particularly important.

Initial exposures might be done from home, like making phone calls to peers; sending texts to relatives, peers, and friends; or calling stores to practice asking questions. But once you get into the swing of things, you as parents will need to play a major role in driving or walking your kids to shopping malls or supermarkets so exposures can be practiced in public settings. In addition, some exposures will need to be done without your real-time participation, like those at school, and kids will need to take the lead. You can approach these by making time together in the evening to set up exposures for the next day and review those completed earlier in the day.

Remember to set up the exposures as an experiment to test the expectations that make the social situations scary. You can refer back to the expectations that you and your child identified in the avoidance cycle. A typical feared outcome we hear all the time in our clinic is *I will mess up and people will judge me.*

It is helpful to be as specific as possible about what your child fears they will do wrong, such as freeze up and not say anything, say the wrong thing, or maybe that other people won't hear them. It is also helpful to be specific about what being judged by others looks like. Ask your child how they will know people are judging them. Would it look like peers rolling their eyes? Making a face? Teasing? Giggling? Turning away? Whispering to a classmate? Imitating in a mocking voice? Walking off? Laughing? Many times, kids aren't sure how they might be judged and equally what it would entail.

So, it helps to set up exposures to test whether they can tolerate the uncertainty of not knowing for sure if they are being judged.

With the groundwork laid, you can now go ahead and complete the setup process by having your child rate how nervous they are that their fear will come true during the exposure.

## STEP 4: DOING SOCIAL ANXIETY EXPOSURES

During exposures, you and your child need to keep paying close attention by frequently having your child re-rate their anxiety about their fear coming true. With social anxiety the timing of that check-in happens most organically after each attempt. If Maria is doing an exposure to asking questions of store clerks, after each store visit her father can ask: *How did that go? How nervous are you to go to the next store and do it again?*

It is important for Maria's father to ask how nervous she is to do it again, because asking *How nervous are you now?* might lead to a lower rating, not because Maria is building confidence but simply because she is out of the distressing social situation.

Similarly, when kids are doing a practice presentation at home, parents can track their anxiety after each run-through. If the school presentation they're practicing takes 3 minutes to give, parents can rate their child's anxiety at the end, and if it's still riding high, have them do the presentation again and again, rating their anxiety after each repetition.

When exposures are conducted together in public settings, like the mall, when you track anxiety, be sure to be discreet. This is a therapeutic activity, and we don't need to bring unwanted attention to working on personal issues.

When kids complete exposures on their own at school or during other activities, it often is not feasible to rate anxiety in the moment, so they will have to reflect on their ratings when they come home and review how it went with you later in the day.

As already established, exposures are more powerful when they are repetitive, so make sure to have your child repeat the same exposure many times, like calling multiple stores and asking *What time do you close today?* or going to a dozen stores in the mall and asking the same question (*When does your summer sale end?*). Some exposures don't suit this so well—like ordering food in a restaurant, because you wouldn't go out for dinner five times in the same evening. For exposures like that, you can encourage your child to start a conversation every time the server comes to the table or to talk to different people throughout the evening, such as a few words checking in with the host or hostess or asking a different server where the bathrooms are.

When anxiety decreases, you want to draw your child's attention to what they are learning. Specifically, that they are talking to people and not making mistakes, or if they do make a mistake, that no one seems to be paying attention.

You also need to keep an eye out for avoidance. For example, your child talking in a very quiet voice, not making eye contact, or gravitating toward people who look more approachable and don't seem in a hurry, like an elderly grandmother, rather than toward kids just a bit older than them who offer more of a challenge. When you notice this, point it out calmly and ask them to do the next repetition without the avoidance.

More so than with other forms of anxiety, the child's fear can sometimes come true with social exposures. Maybe the sales assistant doesn't respond to Maria's question about where the scarves are because Maria spoke so quietly they didn't hear her, or the clerk in the clothing store is visibly impatient due to understaffing that day and snaps at Maria. Should this happen, it can feel like your child's worst nightmare coming true, and they understandably feel judged and upset.

In response, try to be as warm and supportive as possible, agree with your child that it was an unpleasant experience, and then prepare to move on to the next repetition of the exposure. Being able to do it again, even after one attempt went poorly, and then being successful is a powerful experience. Fortunately, negative reactions from others are infrequent, and kids are mostly going to be surprised by how friendly people are.

Social exposures are nevertheless challenging and may require a good deal of parental patience. While your child is walking around the mall, waiting for the perfect person to approach, your frustration can build as he or she passes up one exposure opportunity after another. It's important to stay calm if this happens, be supportive, and warmly praise your child for each attempt they do muster the courage to make.

If needed you can also, in a firm but calm manner, remind your child that you both have a limited amount of time to complete the exposure, and if they have not approached someone in 5 minutes, you will have to try again later, and they will have the previously agreed consequences for an incomplete exposure. It may feel like you're being overly harsh, but part of being supportive is also providing firm expectations that motivate kids to work hard.

## STEP 5: ENDING A SOCIAL ANXIETY EXPOSURE

The general goal for social anxiety exposures is for your child to learn that certain social situations don't go as poorly as their anxiety had them believe they would. This means they come to the realization that they are much less likely to make mistakes than they thought. And when they do make a mistake, sometimes on purpose, sometimes by accident, nobody seems to mind or is actually paying that much attention.

That being said, social anxiety exposures can never really prove or disprove the main fear driving social anxiety, which is that people will judge them. Yes, we have had a good conversation about what signs to look for that people are being judgmental: whether that's an eye roll, a rude comment, or a curt response. But we all also know that people can act politely even if they are very upset or annoyed with us and mask their anger or irritation. For these reasons, a third goal for social anxiety exposures is for your child to learn that they can handle not knowing for sure whether they are being judged. A social anxiety exposure can end when these goals have been met.

Applying our general rule of thumb, your child should continue repeating the exposure activity until their anxiety has come down by half. If Maria begins her exposure to asking store clerks for scarves with an anxiety rating of 6, she should continue until her anxiety about asking the next clerk is running at a 3 or less.

This is no hard-and-fast rule, so if this is the first try at a challenging exposure or if you have simply run out of stores to go to, the exposure might end with anxiety still running higher than half. If Maria can say that her anxiety has come down at least a little and she is able to handle it, even though it stayed high, that is still success. In addition, we would like her to be able to say to her parents something along the lines of *My fear did not come true, I didn't make mistakes, and even when the salesclerk didn't hear me the first time, she was still really nice when I had to repeat myself.* Most importantly, we want Maria to leave the exposure saying she is willing to do that exposure again or that she feels ready to handle that social situation in her everyday life.

## STEPS 6 AND 7: REPETITION AND WORKING IN THE MOMENT WITH SOCIAL ANXIETY

Learning to feel more confident in social situations takes practice. Most kids are in many social situations every day, and if they are shy and nervous they are probably doing a lot of avoidance to cope. That continued frequent avoidance maintains fear and worry. This means that kids, with parent coaching, need to do not only planned exposures but also small on-the-fly exposures that replace moments of avoidance with interactions. This usually takes conscious effort by both the child and their parents.

## PARENTS' ROLE WHEN WORKING ON SOCIAL ANXIETY

Parents need to be particularly active helping their kids with social anxiety exposures. Social exposures frequently take more time and effort to plan and do because you are dependent on other people being available or going to public places. This organizing typically falls to parents. On the other hand, the ability of parents to directly coach and assist with exposures is more limited, especially with teenagers whose social interactions almost exclusively occur outside the parents' presence. Parents still need to help, by planning exposures for the next day and reviewing progress afterward, as well as making arrangements for kids to be in social situations, such as signing kids up for activities or setting an expectation that teens will attend the school pep rally.

## COMMON CHALLENGES WITH SOCIAL ANXIETY

Likely the most common challenge will revolve around the logistics of planning. How do you find kids for your child to talk with and practice on? This involves setting things up well and choosing locations where exposures can be overseen—any location where young people and kids go outside of school, such as a park, a playground, the mall, or the gym at the fitness club. Despite these efforts, designing realistic exposures that bring on your child's anxiety can be a challenge, especially if your child is almost exclusively nervous with peers they see regularly. Our goal then would be to treat planned exposures as practice and emphasize supporting them to do on-the-fly exposures on their own during school or other activities.

## TRACKING PROGRESS ON SOCIAL ANXIETY

Our end goal for social anxiety exposures is not to turn shy and quiet children into social butterflies but to raise a child's confidence and comfort levels so they can do the things they need to do in their everyday lives. We would like for them to be able to function in social settings without distress or avoidance—make conversations at family gatherings, answer questions in class, speak confidently with an adult authority figure, make small talk in a store, and catch up with peers at school over lunch.

More concretely, a sign of progress may be when your child, potentially with your encouragement, signs up for an extracurricular activity or attends school events that social anxiety has long prevented them from doing or joining. Overall success would be when the concerns that led you and your child to start exposure therapy have improved. This might include your child no longer resisting going to school, avoiding clubs or activities, staying home alone all weekend, or looking to you to talk for them in restaurants and other public places.

If, however, despite your best efforts, your child is not progressing and remains overly distressed in social situations, then I would suggest it's time to seek out further professional help. One advantage of the program at our clinic is that by working in groups, we have a ready set of participants for social anxiety exposures.

# 11

# Exposure Therapy for Generalized Anxiety Disorder

Generalized anxiety disorder (or GAD) is not tied to any one situation or theme. Children with general anxiety tend to worry most days about many things. All that worry begins to affect how kids feel physically and gets in the way of doing daily activities.

When considering whether GAD best describes your child's worries, it's particularly important to make sure that what your child is experiencing is not a response to a stressful situation. With GAD, children worry about situations that will most likely turn out fine—they worry about getting into college even though they get straight As, or they worry about a parent's health even though they are fit and healthy. By contrast, with situational stress, kids are nervous and worried about things that are objectively not going well, so they may rightly worry about their grades because they are failing a few classes. Or they are worrying about their parent's health after a cancer scare. When the situation merits worry, the solution is not for your child to be less worried but to take actions to address the situation, such as tutoring to improve grades or receiving emotional support during a parent's medical treatment.

When fears and worries continue without any evidence that things will go poorly, it may be GAD. This chapter details the use of exposure for varied and shifting worries and anxiety, the approach taken with 16-year-old Kara, whose many worries, especially about doing well enough at school, torment her despite being a highly accomplished and successful young woman.

## STEP 1: BUILDING FROM THE GENERALIZED ANXIETY AVOIDANCE CYCLE

A successful exposure plan needs to be individually tailored to your child's fears and worries, and that process begins with your child's avoidance cycle.

### What sets off generalized anxiety

First, we need to identify what sets off your child's anxiety. We learned earlier that a child's fears and worries can be set off by three different things: activities and situations in the world around them, thoughts they have in their head, and feelings in their body. With GAD the anxiety cycle is mostly set off by thoughts, although those thoughts may be more likely to happen in certain situations.

General worries are usually about things that may happen in the future or have happened in the past, rather than what is going on right now. For example, Kara worries about failing her upcoming math test, not graduating high school, being unable to get into college, never getting a job, and ending up homeless.

All of these events would be unpleasant and very stressful if they happened. But Kara's problems with anxiety are not caused by failing tests or heading toward homelessness, because those things aren't happening. Instead, her anxiety occurs when she simply thinks about those things happening. So, it is the worry thoughts themselves that set off her anxiety.

Within this, it's important to also pay attention to situations and physical feelings that may set off general anxiety. Kara may tend to worry about getting into college mostly when she is sitting at her desk doing homework. Or she may worry excessively about her mom's health after reading a story about breast cancer online. The same could be true for physical feelings. Kara may worry about the possibility of having a brain tumor when she gets a headache.

## Expectations that make generalized anxiety scary

Once you've identified the things that set off your child's anxiety, you next need to pinpoint the expectations that cause your child to feel more nervous about these things than other kids. Separating expectations from the thoughts that set off anxiety can be challenging with GAD because both take place in the child's mind. For this reason, it can be tricky to separate the initial fear-provoking worry (e.g., *I will fail this test*) from the expectation that makes that safe thought scary (e.g., *My worries about failing the test will probably come true*). As with other anxiety disorders, expectations that make worry thoughts seem scary fall into two categories: *something bad will happen* and *I can't handle these fears and worries.*

Because we have identified worries about something bad happening as the thought that sets off anxiety, the expectation that makes that thought scary is *My worry is likely to come true.*

Many kids may have a thought while studying along the lines of *I don't get this topic, I am going to fail this test and I'll stay in high school forever.* However, by the time they plow on and get a handle on the material, those bad events seem unlikely to ever happen and soon enough the child moves on and never gets overly upset. However, when Kara has these thoughts, she believes there is a good chance that the terrible outcomes might happen, and she gets stuck in worry and anxiety.

Another way to approach expectations that often translate more easily to setting up exposures is to focus on kids' confidence that they can handle their worries. For instance, Kara might be able to say, *I know I probably won't fail and be homeless, but it's better to be safe than sorry.* In other words, Kara feels like she can't handle the possibility that she might do poorly. So, we might describe the expectations that make her worry thoughts scary as a case of *I can't handle not knowing for sure that things will turn out okay.*

### Avoidance of generalized anxiety

Next, we need to identify what avoidance strategies your child uses to stay away from the thoughts and situations they fear and, in doing so, denying themselves the opportunity to learn that these thoughts and situations are not as bad as they expect them to be.

Avoidance in GAD generally involves efforts by kids to convince themselves that their worries won't come true. This often takes the form of reassurance seeking or frequently asking parents whether things will be okay. Kara may ask her mom if she is healthy and feeling okay. Or if her dad will be okay driving to work in the pouring rain. When her mom assures her that everything is okay, Kara trusts her opinion and experiences some relief, but soon enough, her nagging worries return and she has to ask again.

Checking is another method of seeking reassurance that worries are not going to come true. Kara might constantly check her grades online to keep reassuring herself that yes, she still has all As. Other children might repeatedly check their backpack to ensure they haven't forgotten to pack their homework. Or check the doors and windows to make sure they are locked, in case someone tries to break in.

Some children avoid any risk that their worries may come true by overpreparing. We saw this with Kara, who spent unnecessary hours on her homework going over the material again and again just to be absolutely sure she understood. She also wrote essay answers that were twice as long as required and did extra credit that wasn't required for classes. All these efforts were designed to reduce that feeling of uncertainty that maybe, just possibly, she might fail a test and never be successful.

Finally, there are children who avoid worry thoughts through distraction. They might read, listen to music, watch a show, or play video games to avoid worrying about failing a test.

## STEP 2: BUILDING FEAR LADDERS FOR GENERALIZED ANXIETY

Drawing up a fear ladder that starts with something easy and progresses up to the very scariest activity works for GAD but may require a few tweaks. You can start by making a list of worries off the top of your child's head and by reflecting back on the topics you recall your child worrying about. The order isn't important at first, as you will next work together on rearranging the worries into a list ordered from least to most distressing. Putting worries in this order might be based on the content of the worry. For example, Kara might be more nervous about academic failure than disappointing her parents. Or it may be that general thoughts about her mother getting sick are easier to handle than specific worries about her mother getting breast cancer.

With this in mind, here is an example of a fear ladder listing frequent GAD worry thoughts to help you get started.

### Worry thoughts

1. I will get in trouble because I am late to class
2. I will forget my homework and get a bad grade

3. Everyone will stop being friends with me
4. Burglars will break into the house
5. I will fail my class
6. My mom is late home from work because she got into an accident
7. My sister will get cancer
8. I will never get a good job because I'm not doing well enough at school
9. My parents will die in a car accident

After making a list tailored to your child's worries, it can be helpful to make a fear ladder of situations and activities that make these worries more realistic and intense. For example, Kara and her parents might list working on school assignments the night before a test as a time when worries about failing are most challenging.

Similar to social anxiety mishap exposures, you can design exposures where your child does something purposely wrong to bring on worry. It could be Kara writing a sloppy homework assignment on purpose, writing the wrong date on another piece of homework, or misspelling her own name or even the teacher's name.

Examples of exposures involving purposely making mistakes that are easier to begin with could be downloading a practice test or worksheet unrelated to your child's classes, having them make deliberate mistakes, and handing the flawed worksheet in to you. To increase realism, if a child has assignments at school that get turned in but are not graded, getting one answer deliberately wrong could be purposely done without the risk of hurting their grade.

Other action or situation exposures could focus on reducing avoidance, such as setting a time limit for homework to prevent excessive overworking or rechecking. Exposures can also be planned ahead of time. For example, Dad purposely coming home later than usual from work can be set up as an opportunity for the child to do a thought exposure about something bad happening to him.

For more general worries about the consequences of making mistakes, your child could do an exposure like riding an elevator, pushing the wrong button and then another wrong button, to test whether other people in the elevator get mad. The goal of all these exposures is to create practice experiences and real-life experiments that bring on their daily worries.

Here is an example of a fear ladder of activities to bring on worry thoughts that you can use as is or tweak to better match your child's fears.

### Activities to bring on worry thoughts

1. Complete a non-school worksheet or test that is too hard for you, have someone grade it, and repeat your worry thoughts
2. Make some mistakes on math problems and let others see them
3. Arrange for a parent to be late, repeat the thought that there has been an accident, and do not call for reassurance
4. Without prearranging, repeat the thought that a parent has been in an accident when they are late and do not call for reassurance
5. Practice making mistakes by writing an illegible word in a note to someone
6. Purposely make errors (e.g., misspellings, poor grammar) on an email that you send to someone
7. Turn in an assignment to someone you know (e.g., a parent) and have them give you a bad grade
8. Purposely make mild errors (e.g., sloppy writing, misspellings, poor grammar) in an assignment or report you are turning in

9. Limit the amount of time that you study for a test or spend on an assignment
10. Arrive late to a class, club, or activity
11. Push the wrong button in the elevator

Another important way to make general worry exposures more challenging is to increase your child's independence in completing them. You can make a third fear ladder that gives structure for how to combine the thought exposures with the worry-provoking situations, with less and less support. Such a list would typically begin with thought exposures—repeating the worry thoughts at a calm, planned time with you. Next, they would repeat the thoughts by themselves, alone at home, without your support. Then they would repeat the thoughts during one of the challenging activities with your support, like repeating worries about failing school after completing homework rather than rechecking it. The penultimate step would be doing thought exposures on their own at a planned time in a challenging situation. And then the final step would be your child doing exposures entirely alone in a challenging situation when it happens, perhaps during lunch at school, when they are worried about the test in their next class.

Here are possible steps you can follow for making a third fear ladder focusing on handling worries with more independence.

### Steps for doing worry exposures with increasing independence

1. Repeat worry thoughts at a calm, planned time with support
2. Repeat worry thoughts at a calm, planned time alone
3. Repeat worry thoughts while doing a planned activity that brings on worries, with support

4. Repeat worry thoughts while doing a planned activity that brings on worries, alone
5. Repeat worry thoughts in the moment when the worries start for real, with support
6. Repeat worry thoughts in the moment when the worries start for real, alone

The format of these three fear ladders, tailored to the content of your child's specific worries, can provide a solid guide to completing exposures for GAD.

## STEP 3: SETTING UP GENERALIZED ANXIETY EXPOSURES

Setting up an exposure for general anxiety begins with you and your child deciding together which worry you are going to work on. The primary fear ladder listing all your child's different worries is your basic guide for deciding what to work on. While some children with GAD get very upset while repeating their worries, regardless of how closely they relate to what's happening in their lives, other kids may say their thoughts only bother them during actual real-life situations. For this reason, rather than following the fear ladder, sometimes the best worry to work on is the one that happens to be most distressing to your child at the moment. While Kara may in general be much more worried about her future success than she is about her mother's health, this might be flipped at the time they've set aside for exposures since her mom just got back from a doctor's appointment for a routine screening. In that case, Kara may decide the health exposure is a more helpful worry to work on at that time.

Thought exposures are usually set up as experiments to test the expectation that these worries are too much to handle and that a child will remain anxious throughout the exercise. We can phrase this prediction as *I won't be able to stop worrying* or *I will eventually break down* or *I won't be able to handle these worries on my own* or *I won't be able to handle my worries unless I do something to fix it.*

As we know, the other expectation is this: *My fear is likely to come true.* Since general worries are often about things that might happen in the future, we usually can't prove or disprove them during an exposure. To make a testable exposure, we might rephrase those predictions as *I can't handle not knowing if my fear will come true* or *I will keep worrying until I know my fear won't come true* or *I will keep believing my fear is likely to come true.*

You can now complete the setup by having your child rate how nervous they are that their fear will come true during the exposure.

## STEP 4: DOING GENERALIZED ANXIETY EXPOSURES

The essence of thought exposures for GAD is identifying the most distressing thought and repeating it over and over again until the emotion is drained from it. The most straightforward way to do this is have your child write the thought down and then repeat it out loud over and over again. The goal is to as accurately as possible capture your child's worry without making it positive or more realistic. If Kara worries she will fail her math test and never get a job, she needs to repeat: *I am going to fail my math test and never get a job.* The advantage of repeating a thought aloud is that, no matter how unpleasant the thought, it will eventually get boring.

Over the years, kids have at times told us that they tend to zone out repeating thoughts out loud and that doing this can feel unrealistic. Another way of doing worry exposures is for kids to repeat the thought silently or to picture or imagine their worry happening. This is a powerful approach to worries, as it is more realistic and often causes more anxiety. That can make it more challenging, and it may take longer for anxiety to decrease, which is fine because it means it is a good learning experience, but it can be hard to stick with. Also, it is harder for you to monitor the exposure as you have no idea if your child is daydreaming, thinking about something else, or dedicatedly repeating the worry thought. To combine the best parts of both approaches, we usually have kids start with an out-loud thought exposure and then progress to imagining it silently for a while and then having them once more repeat it out loud. Having them alternate back and forth helps you supervise their efforts.

Two final methods, as we looked at earlier, can be writing down the thought and reading it over and over again. And more abstract, but occasionally the best way, is having you as their parent say the worry thought over and over again for them.

In the end the best approach to worry exposures is the one that is the most realistic to your child's fear and that brings on the most anxiety. Figure out with your child what you need to do to be as realistic as possible and then experiment with different approaches until you find the one that works best.

While your child is repeating their worry thoughts, you can track their anxiety by periodically asking, *How nervous are you now?* or *How nervous are you to continue?* The main thing we want to avoid when tracking anxiety during thought exposures is asking or having kids respond about how nervous they would be if the feared situation were happening. The events kids are worrying about would mostly be bad if they happened, and we don't expect that to change just by them sitting and thinking about it happening. Also, with general worry, the problem is not Kara being nervous when she fails a test, the problem is that she gets acutely nervous just *thinking* about failing a test. So, the anxiety ratings need to focus on how your child feels in the moment repeatedly focusing on their worry.

During the exposure, you should be on the lookout for avoidance. Sometimes kids start to avoid the exposure by turning the thought into something more positive. Kara might say: *I am worried that I will fail the test, but that is silly because I have studied.* Rather than being an exposure to a feared thought, this statement is providing reassurance and helping her avoid her fear. In this case, Kara's mother would encourage her to focus on the fear and repeat the thought: *I will fail the test.*

### STEP 5: ENDING A GENERALIZED ANXIETY EXPOSURE

You will know a general worry exposure is complete when your child says the thought has become boring and that they don't need to do anything to get reassurance. The goal for Kara would be for her to say she is feeling calm enough to put her homework away without rechecking again for mistakes. By and large, the most important lesson kids are learning from worry thought exposures is that their anxiety goes down even if they focus on their worry and even if nobody reassures them everything will be okay. In this sense, general worry exposure is often about handling not knowing things for certain, and we find that as kids' anxiety comes down through repeating the scary thought, they start to believe their worries less. So, although Kara has not learned anything new about her test or how she will do, she is less convinced that she will fail, simply because her fear has drained away, allowing her to think more clearly and calmly about what is realistic and what isn't.

### STEPS 6 AND 7: REPETITION AND WORKING IN THE MOMENT WITH GENERALIZED ANXIETY

More than with other forms of anxiety, planned exposures are mostly an opportunity to learn and practice a new approach to worries. And the important work is kids and parents applying this strategy in times of real worry. Kara may never find planned exposures very challenging. The process of selecting a worry from the list, doing some practice assignment, and repeating the thoughts may always feel safe and structured and without real consequences. The real value of these exercises, though, is that now she and her parents know what to do when her worries strike for real. The next time Kara resists unwinding with her parents before bed because she wants to put excessive, out-of-proportion finishing touches to her homework, her parents can use that as an opportunity to bring in an exposure. They may have her repeat: *My teacher will be disappointed in my work* over and over until her anxiety lowers enough that she can see the moment as it really is, pack up her books, and go downstairs to join the family game night.

## PARENTS' ROLE WHEN WORKING ON GENERALIZED ANXIETY

As always, you will be in charge of taking the lead and ensuring that planned exposures are arranged and completed. Perhaps more importantly with general worries, you will need to proactively intervene and lead on-the-fly exposures when worries actually distress your child in the moment. This can look like noticing when your child is struggling to handle anxiety on their own, as in Kara refusing to stop studying before bed. Or it can take the form of you responding to requests for reassurance with a prompt to do an exposure.

If Kara asks her mother for the second time that evening, *Mom, your doctor's appointment went well, right, and nothing was wrong?*, rather than providing reassurance her mother can say, *That sounds like worrying, I think this is a good time to do a thought exposure, do you need my help?* To which Kara can respond, *No, I can do it* and proceed to repeat out loud, *My mom is sick and dying* over and over until she no longer feels the need for her mother's reassurance.

Although you will play an important and leading role in helping your kids use exposure to break free from worrying, you will also need to fade into the background to promote independence. Seeking reassurance is a primary form of avoiding general worries, and your mere presence during exposures can signal to your child that there is nothing to worry about. It is best to do exposures together so both of you learn how it works first. Then, once your child understands the process, they can do exposures by themselves and tell you how it went afterward. Eventually, when they are doing on-the-fly exposures to everyday anxieties, they can report they handled their worries independently without sharing the nature of the worry itself.

## COMMON CHALLENGES WITH GENERALIZED ANXIETY EXPOSURES

Admittedly, thought exposures are a strange beast. Many of us today are familiar with the idea of the power of positive thinking and upbeat affirmations, so repeating negative, distressing thoughts seems at first entirely counterintuitive. Add to this the general fact that exposures by design make kids feel more nervous before they begin to feel confident, and it can seem very challenging for you and your child to embrace thought exposures.

For these reasons, we usually recommend that families do their first thought exposures in the clinic with us to learn how it goes before trying it on their own. If you don't have a therapist to work with, you might start by repeating worry thoughts unrelated to a specific anxiety to try it out. Back in the day, to calm our 5th-grader nerves before free throws, my elementary school basketball coach told us to repeat the word *asparagus* over and over because it would quickly become ridiculous and we'd end up grinning and feeling more at ease.

On the flip side, you don't need to make your child's worry even worse via a negative tweak in the other direction. If kids are bothered by really scary worries, we do need to have them repeat those, but we don't need to make up worse thoughts just to amplify their worries.

Imperfection around schoolwork presents another common challenge when working on general worries. There can be a fine line between healthy anxiety, concern, and motivation that drives kids to be responsible, successful students and excessive worry about perfection that can make life difficult. Our goal is to help your child be happy and successful, not bring down their grade point average. So while it's important to do exposures involving being imperfect by making small mistakes with schoolwork or limiting the length of answers or time spent studying, we don't want to do an exposure that would actually lower a student's grades.

## TRACKING PROGRESS ON GENERALIZED ANXIETY

Our goal for GAD exposures is for kids to feel more confident that they can handle everyday worries. We don't expect or want to erase worry altogether, because worrying is a natural and important response to stressful or challenging situations. What we do want is for excessive worries to no longer cause problems. So, when looking for signs of success, we often reflect back to the concerns that led us to seek help. For Kara's parents, that would mean asking: Is she going to bed at a decent time and spending time with the family? Does she appropriately limit the time she spends on homework? Has she stopped asking for reassurance about the health of her family members? Has she skipped an opportunity for extra credit so she can hang out with friends on the weekend?

If you are not seeing improvement or if the concept of repeating worry thoughts seems too strange to supervise on your own, don't worry. The next step is to seek out a therapist specializing in anxiety who can help you and your child launch exposure therapy.

# 12

# Exposure Therapy for Separation Anxiety Disorder

Separation anxiety disorder is when children feel very nervous or afraid of being away from their parents. Although these fears are fairly common for young children first going off to school, for some kids the anxiety worsens over time and spreads to other situations, such as bedtime. When fear and worry begin to interfere with age-appropriate daily activities like staying home alone, being dropped off at gymnastics, sleeping in their own bed, or playing in the living room while parents are making dinner, that crosses a line to being separation anxiety disorder.

As with other anxiety disorders, before we settle into work on separation anxiety, we need to make sure we are addressing the correct problem. If being separated from you makes your child nervous, you will see that anxiety appear no matter where they or you are going. However, if your child is only afraid to separate for a single activity, like going into school, but not going over to a friend's house or being home alone, then it may be anxiety about that situation, like social anxiety around kids at school, or they may be experiencing a stress in that situation, such as academic difficulties or being bullied.

For yet other kids, fear of separation may be a reaction to stress at home, such as a parent's illness or extended absence due to work or military deployment, or perhaps arguing and fighting at home. In these cases, it might be more appropriate to address the underlying challenges or help the child cope with difficulties that can't be avoided.

As we move through how to plan and do separation anxiety disorder exposures, we're going to catch up with Alex, whose fear of being away from his parents interferes with going to school, staying with a babysitter while Mom and Dad go on a date night, and even sleeping in his own bed unaccompanied.

## STEP 1: BUILDING FROM THE SEPARATION ANXIETY AVOIDANCE CYCLE

A successful exposure plan needs to be individually tailored to the fears and worries that make separation challenging for your child. And that process starts with looking at your child's avoidance cycle.

### What sets off separation anxiety

First, we need to identify what sets off your child's anxiety. Separation anxiety is primarily set off by situations that require your child to be away from you as a parent. Common examples include: the child being left alone in their bedroom at night, being dropped off at school, being left at sports practice or dance class, being left with a babysitter while the parents go to a friend's birthday party, or spending the night at the grandparents'. Some children, particularly younger children, may even become upset simply being out of eyesight from a parent and will follow them around the house, pounding on the bathroom door when separated for the briefest moment. For older kids, there are many activities that require independence that might set off their anxiety, such as using a public bathroom, going into a store alone, walking the dog, or waiting in the car while Mom runs into a convenience store to grab a carton of milk. In addition to these situations, separation anxiety can also be set off by thoughts. Typically, these thoughts center around something bad happening to a parent or to the child themselves and tend to trend toward any theme that says their parents won't come back. These thoughts usually, but not always, cause anxiety only during times of separation. They are generally less important for identifying what sets off your child's anxiety and typically fit more with the expectations that make separation scary. However, we sometimes include thought exposures in our treatment plans at the clinic, so it is helpful to consider and factor in anxiety-provoking thoughts when putting together the avoidance cycle.

### Expectations that make separation scary

Now that we have identified the situations that set off your child's anxiety, we can move on to understanding what your child expects will happen that makes appropriate levels of independence and time away from you as their parents so frightening.

Since separation anxiety occurs most often in younger children, it is not unusual for young kids to have difficulty articulating what they expect to happen. Some kids may simply say: *I don't know* or *I miss my parents.* These reactions fall more in the *I can't handle being away from my parents* category. However, often kids do expect something bad to happen, such as: *My parents won't come back, My parents will get hurt, I won't know what to do, Nobody will be there to help me feel better,* or *Someone will take me.*

Sometimes at the clinic we ask some of these thoughts to do double duty, since they set off anxiety and serve as expectations that make separation scary. For example, we might say playing in a room alone makes a child nervous because they expect their parents will leave and never come back. Or we could say that thinking about their parents leaving and not coming back makes a child nervous because they expect they can't handle that thought on their own. There is no right answer, and we shouldn't get too caught up splitting hairs. What's important is that we are thinking about how your child reacts to both situations *and* thoughts in a way that makes them nervous.

### Avoidance of separation situations

Next, we need to identify what avoidance strategies your child uses to prevent separation and, in doing so, miss out on the opportunity to learn that being independent is not as overwhelming as they expect it to be.

The most visible way that kids practice avoidance when they have separation anxiety is by becoming very upset and clinging to their parents. This clinging, crying, becoming upset, or whining often delays separation and, at least at first, elicits a reassuring response from parents.

Avoidance may also continue after separation through calling out to parents from behind the door, waving in a distressed manner as parents pull out of the driveway, making phone calls to check on them, or sending panicky text messages.

When kids feel scared and overwhelmed by separation, any parental comfort and warm caretaking or response to calls or texts provides immediate, if short-lived, relief. Moreover, while crying and clinging typically does not result in avoiding their being dropped off at school, it may prevent future separation as parents decide their child is not ready to join other activities, be left with a sitter, or sleep alone.

---

When Alex and his parents sat down to fit his experience into the avoidance cycle, they decided most situations where he was separated from his parents set off his anxiety, the most intense and frequent being going to school in the morning and going to sleep in his own bed alone at night and, running a close third, any attempt by his parents to leave him at home with a sitter.

Working together, they identified that he expected that while his parents were gone, he would start to miss them straightaway and nobody else but them could help him feel better. To avoid separation, they noted that Alex refused to sleep on his own and would come out or call out if his parents tried to leave him; that when his mom tried to run any errand without him, he'd cling to her at the front door and cry; and that he sought multiple reassurances that his dad would pick him up on time before getting out of the car at school.

## STEP 2: BUILDING SEPARATION ANXIETY FEAR LADDERS

Now that we have used the avoidance cycle to organize your child's separation anxiety, let's use the identified items that set off anxiety to build fear ladders for your child. Separation anxiety is most often set off by situations and activities, and therefore most exposures on a fear ladder will be action exposures.

When building fear ladders for separation anxiety, we typically have three main considerations. First, we need to primarily focus on directly practicing the act of separating and being away from parents in increasingly challenging situations. Second, it is often helpful to add in exposures to help your child learn they can handle scary thoughts related to separation. And finally, we usually need to clearly set goals to decrease the anxious behaviors (crying and clinging) that typically occur during separation so your child can separate from you with increasing levels of calmness.

With those principles in mind, difficulties with separation anxiety generally fall into three categories that can translate into their own fear ladders. The first place to start is separating and being alone, away from you, in your home. If your child is too nervous to play in a room alone while you go to the bathroom, it is going to be very hard to work on separation with a sitter or going to school. The basic goal of this ladder is to break the avoidance cycle in which your child previously earned your soothing support through acting anxious, by instead rewarding and encouraging your child's calm independence with your warm attention and praise. More concretely, explain to your child that if they are playing calmly in the room alone, you will check in often to see how they are doing, but if they get upset and call out, you will wait until they are quiet before checking on them. To move up the fear ladder, we make the exposure more difficult by checking in less frequently or having your child stay in a more challenging situation. Here is an example of a fear ladder to encourage being alone at home (each item should only be attempted if age-appropriate).

### Separating from parents at home

1. Repeat scary thoughts with a parent
2. Stay in a room alone with a parent checking in every few minutes if calm and quiet
3. Stay in a room alone and repeat scary thoughts with a parent checking in if calm and quiet
4. Stay in a room alone repeating scary thoughts with long breaks between parent check-ins
5. Stay upstairs or downstairs alone and repeat scary thoughts with a parent checking in if calm and quiet
6. Stay in a very challenging room (like with the lights out or with parents outside in the yard) alone and repeat scary thoughts with check-ins
7. Separate calmly when parents go outside the house (like to get the mail)

8. Stay home alone for a short time while parents walk around the block
9. Stay home alone for 30–60 minutes while parents run a short errand
10. Stay home alone for a few hours while parents go out for dinner
11. Stay home alone without knowing where parents are going or when they will be back

Once your child is able to separate during the day and you and your child understand how to use parental check-ins to encourage calm, quiet independence, we can shift our focus to issues after dark. You will notice that we hold off on expecting kids to stay in bed and put themselves back to sleep in the middle of the night until they have the confidence to go to bed alone at bedtime. If your child feels nervous at bedtime because of worry or scary thoughts, it might be helpful to practice some thought exposures during the day so they are prepared to handle those worries independently at bedtime. As with the fear ladder for exposures focused on separation at home, the key to encouraging kids to stay in bed quietly is to check on them while they are calm, before they have a chance to call out in fear.

Here is a sample fear ladder for exposures to your child staying in their own bed, by themselves, at bedtime.

### Sleeping alone

1. Repeat scary thoughts with a parent
2. Stay in bed at bedtime with a parent checking in if calm and quiet (parents can help repeat scary thoughts if needed)
3. Stay in bed at bedtime with a parent checking in if calm and quiet (repeat scary thoughts alone if needed)

4. Stay in bed at bedtime without a parent checking in (repeat scary thoughts alone if needed)
5. If child wakes in the middle of the night, return to bed with parent checking in if calm and quiet (parents can help repeat scary thoughts if needed)
6. If child wakes in the middle of the night, do not get parents and stay in bed alone

Older kids who have separation anxiety may be more likely to feel nervous in public settings that require age-appropriate independence. So here is a sample fear ladder to guide exposures for practicing independence in public (each item should only be attempted if age-appropriate).

### Separating in public

1. Practice sitting by oneself in a familiar place, like a therapist's waiting room
2. Walk around a familiar place alone, like the floor the therapist's office is situated on
3. Walk around in public alone
4. Ride elevators to another floor alone
5. Find your way to a place alone
6. Go to a friend's house without a parent
7. Play at a park away from a parent
8. Go somewhere with a friend and their parents
9. Walk into a store alone while parent waits outside
10. Go into public restrooms alone

Sometimes after increasing a child's confidence being alone at home, it is necessary to have a specific plan to translate these gains to separating at school. A school-focused fear ladder to help Alex return to school might start with his mother walking him all the way into school and dropping him off at the classroom or school counselor's office. For the next step, his mother might drop him off at the school's entrance and wait as he walks in alone. From there, Alex might say good-bye to his mother in the car and walk in by himself.

These fear ladders, with any adaptations needed to best speak to your child's fears, form the foundation of your separation anxiety exposure plan. Not all kids will feel anxious or need to practice each of the three situations. The decision to add repeating scary thoughts to the action-oriented exposures should be based on your child's needs. Younger children who don't have clear fears of something bad happening may have difficulty understanding and frequently don't need the addition of thought exposures.

## STEP 3: SETTING UP SEPARATION ANXIETY EXPOSURES

The essence of most separation anxiety exposures, particularly those revolving around practicing being alone in a room or in bed, involves you as the parent using your attention to encourage brave behavior in your child.

Setting up an exposure begins with you and your child choosing an activity from a fear ladder. Part of setting the degree of difficulty involves deciding what situation the child will be in. Are they sitting in the living room or upstairs? Where will you be, in the next room or on a different floor?

Next, what is the child expected to be doing during the exposure? Can they be playing, which is a distraction? Playing will make the exposure easier through avoidance, but it is often appropriate to allow if your child is still very young. Alternatively, will your child be expected to focus on the exposure by repeating scary thoughts, an additional challenge when needed and age-appropriate?

Finally, you need to decide in advance how often you will be checking in on your child. Earlier exposures on the fear ladder, when children are pretty nervous and just learning they can be successful, will need parents checking in frequently. After some success, a more challenging exposure will start to see you as a parent come in less often. Agreeing on a plan during setup for each of these aspects, as much as the age of your child affords, will help both you and your child be successful.

Next, we need to set the exposure up as an experiment. Separation exposure often tests the expectation that kids won't be able to handle being alone. Children expect to stay nervous until they are reunited with their parents. If kids have other fears, such as *My dad won't come back* or *Somebody will take me,* write those down too. You can now complete the setup by having your child rate how nervous they are to do the exposure.

## STEP 4: DOING SEPARATION ANXIETY EXPOSURES

As for all exposures, you as parent will check in periodically to have your child re-rate their anxiety. However, during separation anxiety exposures this check-in takes on extra importance because the check-in is an opportunity for parents to give warm attention, and the time between check-ins is part of the degree of difficulty.

So, Alex's mother might start his exposure to staying in bed by getting his initial anxiety rating and then saying, *I know this is hard so I will check on you frequently if you are quiet.* She then steps out of the room, counts to ten, steps back in and says, *You're doing a great job, how nervous are you to keep doing this?* Since he just started the exposure, his anxiety hasn't changed yet, so his mom replies: *Keep it up. I'll check in again soon as long as you're quiet.* She then waits 30 seconds, steps back in, and says the same thing again.

The goal here is for Alex's mother to check on him before he has an opportunity to act on his anxiety by calling out or leaving his room. Gradually, she increases the amount of time between check-ins, and Alex gradually learns a new routine where he gets attention and praise for staying in bed quietly by himself, not for acting upset and calling out. Along the way he also learns that sleeping alone is not so scary and he can handle it.

This method of parents checking in to give positive attention and having their child re-rate their anxiety can be used for many of the exposures in the above fear ladders. You can use this approach with an exposure to your child being alone in the living room while you step out to another room. And also as you increase the challenge to your child being upstairs in their bedroom while you remain downstairs.

A next level of difficulty could be for you to not check in at all during the exposure. In this case your child would rate their anxiety on their own, or you could simply review their recall of ratings at the end. This would be the approach to use for exposures to staying home alone, such as when you walk around the block.

One natural way to up the level of challenge when staying home alone is to extend the length of time that you are away. After an exposure to you taking a walk around the block, you might next run a short errand to pick up dry cleaning and progress to an extended trip to the grocery store and pharmacy. When using time-sensitive goals, it is best not to set a specific time limit, such as five minutes. This can lead kids to focus on just getting through the fixed amount of time knowing that relief is coming at a certain moment regardless of what they do, rather than accepting that they don't know exactly when you will return and that the exposure will not be done until they believe they can handle this level of separation. Instead, stick with general durations in terms of the activity, a walk around the block, or a window of time, such as 20 to 30 minutes and so on.

When separation exposures involve small actions, like riding an elevator to another floor away from their parents, these need to be repeated multiple times. Each time your child returns you can ask: *How nervous are you to do it again?* And off they go again, riding the elevator to a higher floor and back alone.

Finally, during thought exposures, kids will likely repeat something along the lines of *My parents won't come back* or *My parents have died in a car accident and I'll never see them again.* During the initial attempts, you'll be right next to your child, coaching them through these unusual first exposures. Every so often you will then check in with *How nervous are you now?* or *How nervous are you to continue?* The child continues with the exposure until the thoughts they are repeating lose their intense emotion and become boring. After achieving success with direct parental support, the next thought exposure can be done with your child sitting in the living room at a calm time, like a quiet Sunday afternoon, with you doing periodic check-ins as described above. As your child learns they can handle scary thoughts alone by repeating them until they get bored, thought exposures can be used along with any of the other steps on the fear ladder.

## STEP 5: ENDING A SEPARATION ANXIETY EXPOSURE

Generally, the goal for separation anxiety exposures is for your child to realize they can feel comfortable in the situation without you. With exposures where you are checking in on your child every so often as they sit alone or where your child is repeating an activity like riding the elevator, you can end the exposure when their anxiety rating about continuing decreases by at least half from the starting point. For exposures in which you leave them home alone while you run an errand or they go off alone to an activity, like a playdate, the exposure is generally over when the activity is over rather than based on anxiety ratings, due to the fact that you're not going to go out and run five errands back-to-back. In either case, you want to wrap up the exposure by reviewing our two core questions with your child, asking them: *Did your fears come true?* and *What happened to your anxiety?*

Typically, the answers to these questions are pretty straightforward. You and your child are sitting there safely together, so they have not been kidnapped, you have not been in an accident, and you have obviously not forgotten about them and never returned. It is fine to approach these questions with a dot of humor, if it feels appropriate, since kids can feel a bit silly at this debrief. Perhaps more important is ensuring that your child realizes that they began to feel calmer and safer while they were alone, before you came back, as this is an essential lesson of separation exposure.

## STEPS 6 AND 7: REPETITION AND WORKING IN THE MOMENT WITH SEPARATION ANXIETY

Typically, repetition within separation exposures is accomplished by your child sitting alone for an extended time, rather than doing something over and over. Thought exposures and activity exposures, like riding the elevator, include more straightforward repetition of an action or thought. Some earlier exposures are practice for more important and challenging exposures. For example, although Alex's parents are mostly concerned about separation at bedtime and school, they decided to first practice the exposure steps during the day at home as preparation, even though it wasn't that challenging for him. If your child's separation anxiety is worse or primarily occurs in public settings, like when being dropped off at school or they have a fear of getting lost in a grocery store, practicing planned exposures at home first before attempting them in public helps build confidence in the process as well as your child's ability to be successful.

## PARENTS' ROLE WHEN WORKING ON SEPARATION ANXIETY

You know by now how important a part of the exposure team you are and rarely more so than when doing exposures for separation anxiety. Throughout this chapter we have highlighted the importance of you as a parent using your attention and support to encourage calm and brave independence, rather than soothing increasingly anxious responses.

Parents often find it helpful to implement other portions of the motivation plan, such as a basic reward system, in addition to using their attention, especially when their children are younger. Even after planned exposures are successful, kids can still be resistant to separation in the actual real-world moment, in which case you can put together a plan to decrease anxious behavior around separation. For example, if your child is crying and clinging and demanding you say goodbye multiple times when you leave for work in the morning, one small first step might be to expect your child to stop physically clinging, but allow them to continue the multiple goodbyes and crying. Once that is accomplished, the next step would be to remove the crying and the final step would be to remove multiple goodbyes so there is only one goodbye. At that point a successful separation will only include your child saying goodbye with a single hug as you head out to work.

Alex's parents might give him a point each time he successfully completes an exposure, like sitting in the living room alone, staying in his bed alone until he falls asleep, or separating without clinging. Once he has 5 or 10 points, he can cash them in for a small reward like a family trip to his favorite pizza restaurant.

On the other hand, you also need to be prepared to respond when your child is upset and not being successful. During exposures, our goal is to check in quickly before kids begin to act upset. But when that doesn't happen, you should wait until your child calms down and then check in. When it's not possible to wait out the crying, you can make it clear to your child that they have a choice to calm themselves and complete the exposure or have the consequence for not being successful, perhaps loss of a toy or screen time, until they have been successful with the next exposure. In either case it is important for you to remain calm (at least outwardly) and be firm but not angry or overly disappointed.

## COMMON CHALLENGES WITH SEPARATION ANXIETY

The most common challenge encountered by parents when working on separation anxiety with their kids is responding to anxious and resistant behavior. When kids are scared, they naturally express those feelings so that their parents help soothe them. If parents aren't responding, kids begin expressing those feelings more loudly to get their parents' attention. So, when parents start expecting kids to face their fears by separating and being independent, a child's first reaction is often to turn up the volume on their anxious behavior. As a result, things might get worse before they get better. The best approach here is to start small with practice exercises that set your child up for success and give lots of immediate warm praise for gradual progress.

The situations in which separation anxiety occurs also present challenges. You don't need me to tell you that mornings and bedtimes can be some of the most stressful times of the day when raising kids. If the idea of repeatedly checking on your child until they fall asleep seems destined to fail or is simply exhausting, you can alter the approach by setting smaller goals. For instance, Alex's mother might explain that if he stays in bed quietly for 15 minutes with (or perhaps without) her checking on him, then she will come in and lie down with him until he falls asleep. In this approach Alex's mother is still rewarding him with her presence for calmly staying in his room alone, but she is not expecting him to do it until falling asleep. With success, the next night she can expect him to wait 20 minutes before she comes in.

## TRACKING PROGRESS ON SEPARATION ANXIETY

It's helpful for you and your child to set the initial goals as simply getting started and working together to complete practice exposures. Even if playing in a room alone is not that big a deal, successfully introducing your child to a new way to gain your attention through independence is an early sign of progress. Once you begin working on more challenging situations, progress will likely come in fits and starts. Successful exposures and calmer, while not perfect, separations in some situations but not others will gradually increase. Although progress in the important areas may sneak up on you, success will likely be more obvious to you than to your child. You will know you have been successful when your child is going off to school, saying a quick goodbye as you head out to work, and allowing you to arrange a sitter for date night without tears.

If applying exposure and a motivation plan to address your child's separation anxiety doesn't feel right or possible, or if you are not seeing success with your efforts, don't hesitate to seek support from a mental health professional.

# 13

# Exposure Therapy for Panic Disorder and Agoraphobia

Panic attacks are sudden episodes of intense fear and physical symptoms like heart pounding, difficulty breathing, shaking, feeling dizzy, or getting nauseous. When kids have panic disorder, these attacks seem to occur for no reason, and kids start to worry about when and where they will have the next one. When kids start to fear and avoid public situations in which they *might* have a panic attack or feel physically anxious, this can turn into a related disorder, agoraphobia.

Before deciding that panic attacks themselves are the problem, it is important to make sure the episodes are not happening for another reason. Panic attacks can occur within other anxiety disorders when kids are doing a feared activity. It's not improbable that Michael might have a panic attack if his neighbor's dog suddenly escapes and bounds across the street into his front yard while he's playing ball. Or Maria might have a panic attack when her new history teacher announces that everyone in class is going to stand up and give a short speech introducing themselves. In these cases, the panic is a result of another fear, like dogs or public speaking, rather than the root problem.

When panic attacks themselves are the source of the problem, you can follow the steps in this chapter to design an exposure plan to help your child break free of their grip. If you recall, 13-year-old Nora is a successful, bright, and well-adjusted teenager who began to avoid leaving the house after experiencing repeated panic attacks.

## STEP 1: BUILDING FROM THE PANIC AVOIDANCE CYCLE

A successful exposure plan needs to be individually tailored to your child's fears. And that process starts with the avoidance cycle.

### What sets off panic and agoraphobia

First, we need to identify what sets off your child's anxiety. As opposed to social anxiety, where fear is set off by the activity of talking to people, or general anxiety, where it is set off by worry thoughts, panic disorder is unique in that fear and worry is set off by the physical symptoms themselves. What happens is that a child begins to feel dizzy or nauseous or their heart skips a beat, and they react to this as a bad sign of something worse to come, which then brings on more sensations and becomes a full-blown panic attack.

Over time, situations also start to set off worry about panic. Having to go to places where panic attacks have occurred before or where it would be particularly difficult to handle a panic attack sets off worry and fear that panic will strike. These situations often involve scenarios where large groups of people are present, like the lunchroom or a shopping mall, or situations that are hard to leave and can feel claustrophobic, like a classroom or the back corner of a popular and crowded restaurant.

### Expectations that make panic attacks scary

Once you've identified the physical feelings and situations that set off your child's anxiety, the next thing to do is pinpoint the expectations that cause your child to be more afraid of panic feelings than other kids.

When a child has panic disorder, their thoughts transform physical symptoms that are otherwise not dangerous into signs that something very bad is going to happen. So, a bit of heart pounding while out walking ignites thoughts like *I'm going to have a heart attack.* Or a wave of dizziness leads to *I'm going to pass out.* Or tightness in the throat and chest is met with *I'm not getting enough oxygen, I can't breathe.* Kids may also have fears that something bad will happen but are less specific and may use phrases like: *Something is wrong with me, I'm going to lose control,* or *I'm going to start crying in front of everyone.* More often, kids react to the physical symptoms of panic with expectations that these feelings are too much to handle. They might say something like *Panic is really terrible, or frightening, or uncomfortable.* Whether kids believe something bad will happen or that they can't handle the attack, these expectations make physical feelings frightening, which leads to more physical feelings and panic.

### Avoidance of panic attacks

Next, we need to identify what your child has been doing to avoid panic feelings that has prevented them from learning these feelings are manageable. Once a child has experienced a panic attack or recurring panic attacks, they may start to avoid places or situations similar to where the attacks happened. If attacks seem to have happened a lot around crowds, they are going to do their best to avoid crowds. They may avoid eating in the lunchroom or going to shopping malls or big events unless a parent is accompanying them. They may also avoid doing activities that bring on physical symptoms, like sports or exercise, because they fear an increased heart rate or that having to catch their breath will lead to a panic attack. Avoidance can also include preparation to prevent or handle a panic if it occurs. Some kids want to have a water bottle with them so they can drink water to reassure themselves that their throat is not closing when they feel like they're going to suffocate. Or they might want you with them whenever they leave the house because they have come to believe that you are the only person who can help them calm down and feel safe. Avoiding situations, relying on parents, or other strategies to handle situations that can't be avoided helps kids feel more comfortable in the moment and keeps them believing that panic attacks are an ever-present danger they need to be constantly prepared for.

---

When going through the avoidance cycle, Nora and her father identified that her anxiety was set off mostly by her heart suddenly pounding and shortness of breath, the two most distressing physical symptoms she noted, as well as the classroom, where these attacks might occur around peers.

Although initially Nora believed that her panic attacks were a sign of a serious medical problem, like a heart attack, after having them for a while and seeing her doctor, her expectations became predominantly about how she couldn't handle having panic attacks in front of others without freaking out or breaking down. To avoid the distress of having panic attacks, she stayed home rather than going shopping or other places, would escape to the bathroom at school, and tried to have a parent with her whenever possible.

## STEP 2: BUILDING PANIC AND AGORAPHOBIA FEAR LADDERS

Based on our understanding of what sets off anxiety around panic attacks, our fear ladders need to address the physical symptoms of the panic attacks themselves and the situations that are avoided because a panic attack might occur. It is helpful to begin fear ladder building by sitting down with your child and writing out a list of all the physical feelings your child experiences during a panic attack. This might include a pounding heart, a tight chest, trouble breathing, sweatiness, shaking, nausea, or dizziness. Once you have that list written out, make a list of exposure exercises that can bring on those feelings. There are four exposure activities we use most commonly at our clinic to bring on symptoms for panic. For each of the following exercises, the goal is to first do it for a short 10 to 15 seconds to test it out and then work up to repetitions of 60 seconds.

### A fear ladder for panic attack feelings

1. Hyperventilate (by breathing deeply without pauses) until general panic-like feelings of dizziness, chest tightness, or tingling occur
2. Breathe through a cocktail straw (holding your nose closed) to generate feelings of shortness of breath and the sense of not getting enough oxygen
3. Spin around in a swivel chair until feelings of dizziness and being unsteady occur
4. Run up and down a flight of stairs until heart rate is elevated to create a racing heart and sweating

With this first fear ladder in place, the next step is to write out a second list of all the activities, places, and situations that your child has been avoiding for fear of having a panic attack. These situations might include shopping malls, hallways between classes, sporting events, restaurants, or the school bus. Then turn that list into a fear ladder by adding in practice steps and combining situations with exercises that bring on panic feelings. The resulting fear ladder might look like this:

### A fear ladder for panic attacks

1. Bring on panic feelings via hyperventilation or breathing through a cocktail straw at home (or in a therapist's office) with support
2. Bring on panic feelings at home (or in a therapist's office) alone
3. Bring on panic feelings at home (or in a therapist's office) and then walk around and talk
4. Do schoolwork after bringing on panic feelings
5. Go outside the home (in public) after bringing on panic feelings
6. Walk around a crowded shopping mall
7. Bring on panic feelings and then walk around a shopping mall
8. Walk through the school hallways at the busiest time between classes
9. Bring on panic feelings and then walk through the hallways at the busiest time between classes
10. Bring on panic feelings and then stand in a crowd at a sporting event

These two fear ladders form the foundation of your exposure plan for panic and agoraphobia. Your child does not have to do all the physical exercises, only those that successfully bring on the feelings they experience during panic attacks. In addition, make sure to include the actual situations that your child fears in the list of activities and places.

With panic disorder, it's best to start out doing interoceptive exposures to bring on a panic attack in a comfortable situation at home. Then you can combine those with doing exposures in feared places and settings such as a crowded mall. If needed, you can also add in working on intrusive thoughts related to the physical symptoms with the goal of learning to cope with the feelings, thoughts, and situations all together. With that in mind, early exposures will probably be to physical feelings that can be accomplished at home, while later on you will have to travel to crowded situations or plan for your child to complete exposures during the school day.

### STEP 3: SETTING UP PANIC EXPOSURES

To set up exposures as experiments, it helps to look back at the avoidance cycle and the expectations that lead to anxiety. Since panic disorder and agoraphobia center on the fear of panic attacks rather than the situation itself, we need to design our exposures to learn whether or not panic is indeed dangerous.

When setting up an exposure to bring on feelings of panic, perhaps through hyperventilation, your child might expect: *I will have a panic attack* or *I will pass out* or *It will just get worse and worse until I stop.* It is not unusual for kids not to expect anything bad will happen during these exposures, just that it will be too uncomfortable to handle. Once you start doing exposures in public places, kids often fear that they will lose control and draw attention to themselves. So, we might set up our experiment to test the beliefs that *I will freak out,* or *I will break down and start crying,* or *I will have to leave the mall to calm down.*

You can then complete the setup by having your child rate how nervous they are that their fear will come true during the exposure. Nora and her father might decide to begin her exposures with hyperventilation at home. Hyperventilation is an excellent place to start because it brings on a broad range of panic-like symptoms.

When setting up the exposure, Nora's father explains that she will breathe deeply without pause, so a little quicker than normal, but not fast. He will demonstrate how to do it first and then Nora will hyperventilate for about 5 seconds. Once she has the hang of it, they plan that she will gradually work her way up to 60 seconds. Nora fears that the exercise will lead to her having a full-blown panic attack and freaking out. She rates her anxiety to get started at a 7 out of 10.

## STEP 4: DOING PANIC EXPOSURES

During panic exposures a good portion of kids' attention needs to focus inward on what is happening with their physical feelings. For this reason, we often ask a few additional questions when coaching through exposures to bodily feelings. First, we want to make sure that the exercise is successfully bringing on symptoms of panic. So, we may ask: *How similar are your feelings right now to how you feel when you're having a panic attack?* At the beginning of an exercise, like hyperventilation, the answer may be *not very similar,* simply because it often takes some time to allow thc panic-likc feelings to build. It's important to stick with it long enough for kids to start experiencing the feelings strongly enough to judge how similar those feelings are to a panic attack.

Once the exercise is up and running and your child is telling you that it is pretty similar to a panic attack, we can stop asking how similar it is and switch to our standard check-in question: *How nervous are you that your fear will come true?* or *How nervous are you to keep doing this?* We keep repeating this question after each 60 seconds of hyperventilation or whichever exposure exercise you are doing.

Sometimes during exposures to panic feelings, kids equate physical discomfort with anxiety, in which case it can be helpful to also ask how uncomfortable they are. When doing exposure to panic feelings, we expect the discomfort to build and build as the exposure continues, because the more you do something, like hyperventilating, the more you feel dizzy, shaky, tingling, tight in the chest, and overall awful. Despite this discomfort, as the exposure continues and nothing bad happens, your child's fear that something bad will happen decreases. If your child is equating physical discomfort with anxiety, those ratings are unlikely to decrease and the exposure won't feel successful. However, when they have the chance to rate physical discomfort and anxiety separately, they can observe their anxiety ratings decrease even as they continue to rate their discomfort as high.

Let's check in again with Nora and her father as they work through their first exposure. After hyperventilating for about 10 seconds, Nora reported that she felt fine but a little light-headed, not too similar to a panic attack. She then hyperventilated for a further 30 seconds, after which she was also feeling a bit shaky, and her heart was starting to beat faster. Not only was this more similar to a panic attack, but her fear that she would have a full-blown panic attack was up to a rating of 8. Despite that, Nora was still willing to keep going and next time hyperventilated for a whole 60 seconds. After this, she informed her father that her heart was now pounding, her arms and legs were shaky and tingly, and she felt like she was about to cry. All of which she felt when she had one of her regular panic attacks at school. At this point it was pretty clear that she had successfully replicated the sensations of a panic attack and her father stopped asking this question.

Nora again hyperventilated for 60 seconds, after which her father asked: *How uncomfortable are you?* To which Nora replied: *Very, I'd say a 9.* And then he asked: *How nervous are you that you will have a panic attack?* To which she replied: *Also a 9.* She then hyperventilated again for 60 seconds. This time she replied to her father's two questions as follows: *I am still very uncomfortable, still a 9, but nothing different is happening, so my anxiety is down to a 7.* As Nora had now separated physical discomfort and anxiety, her father stopped asking about the discomfort, and they continued Nora's hyperventilating and exclusively rated anxiety.

### STEP 5: ENDING A PANIC EXPOSURE

The goal for panic exposures is to learn that while panic symptoms are very uncomfortable, they are ultimately not dangerous and your child can handle experiencing them. If kids can stick with an activity until their anxiety can be measured as zero, that's amazing, but if it goes down by half, that's good enough. When wrapping up an exposure, it can be helpful to emphasize how uncomfortable and similar to a panic attack the feelings were, in addition to asking our standard questions about fears coming true and what happened to their anxiety levels. Ideally, we would like for Nora to say, *Even though the panic feelings stayed high, nothing bad happened, I didn't have a full panic attack, I didn't start crying, and my fear came down.*

### STEPS 6 AND 7: REPETITION AND WORKING IN THE MOMENT WITH PANIC AND AGORAPHOBIA

As with all exposures, kids often need to repeat a given exposure multiple times before they feel confident they could handle those panic feelings in the moment. Before moving from the initial exercises to bring on panic feelings to exposures in challenging settings, it may be necessary to explore a number of different approaches to fully replicate your child's panic attacks.

Nora might share with her father that although reasonably authentic to a real panic attack at school, the hyperventilation didn't bring on the terrifying feeling that she couldn't get enough air into her lungs. In that case, she and her father would follow the same steps above with breathing through a cocktail straw. Cocktail straws are very narrow and breathing through one brings on the very uncomfortable feeling of not being able to breathe properly. Alternatively,

Nora might need to do an exposure to running up and down the stairs to get her heart really pounding and feeling hot. After experimenting with these activities individually, Nora might combine them, such as hyperventilating until she feels shaky and tingly and then breathing through a cocktail straw to bring on the sensations of running out of air.

Once kids have learned that the physical feelings of panic are not dangerous, the next step is to learn they can function, particularly in real-world situations, while having these feelings. This might begin with standing and walking around, or doing math problems, or giving a speech. Then continue with going out into crowded busy places. Some kids fear simply being in public places even without panic symptoms, so exposures can begin with just going into those situations without additional exercise to bring on panic.

## PARENTS' ROLE WHEN WORKING ON PANIC AND AGORAPHOBIA

Your role when working on panic is the same as standard exposure coaching for all anxiety disorders and OCD. While preferably collaborating with your child, you are in charge when it comes to ensuring that exposures are planned and completed. As long as you are physically healthy—check with your family doctor if you're not sure about this—I think it is helpful for you to do the exercises to bring on panic symptoms with your child too. You don't have to stick it out for the full 60 seconds of hyperventilating, but if you do the first 15- or 30-second trials alongside your child, it will give you a better feel for how hard your child is working and at the same time show your support by not asking them to do anything that you won't do yourself.

As a tricky caveat, like for other disorders, your presence during exposures may interfere with your child having the opportunity to learn they can handle the exposures independently. To address this, after success with directly parent-coached exposures, you and your child can then plan exposures that your child completes on their own, for example, hyperventilating in a room alone, walking away from you in a mall, or bringing on panic symptoms before going to a class at school.

## COMMON CHALLENGES WITH PANIC AND AGORAPHOBIA EXPOSURES

The first common challenge is ensuring that panic disorder is the most accurate description for what your child is experiencing. At our clinic, we see kids with panic disorder or agoraphobia far less frequently than children with other anxiety disorders.

Rather than being primarily afraid of having panic attacks, as in panic disorder, kids more often are having anxiety and panic attacks in response to a situation that frightens them, like public speaking, separating from their parents, or encountering a dog, as in Michael's case. For these children, we need to do exposures to the feared activity or situation itself, rather than to panic feelings.

When kids do have panic disorder, another challenge you may run into is the difficulty of bringing on realistic panic symptoms. Children might say it feels similar but it's not frightening because they know why it's happening. *But Mom, when I have a panic attack in real life, I don't know why it's happening and that's what makes it scary.* That's an insightful and reasonable thought. In response, it can be helpful to explain that all planned exposures are practice and that it is always more challenging in the moment. If the physical feelings are the same, or at least similar, the more kids practice handling them during exposures, the more likely they will be to successfully handle the real symptoms when they strike them at school or elsewhere.

## TRACKING PROGRESS ON PANIC AND AGORAPHOBIA

As with other anxiety disorders, success when working on panic disorder comes in stages. Simply finding exposure exercises that accurately mimic panic attacks is an early sign that you are on the right track. Completing your first exposure to hyperventilation or other exercises and watching as your child realizes *Yes, that was miserably uncomfortable, but I am just not scared anymore,* is an inspiring milestone.

Ultimately, as with all anxiety disorders, the goal is to get kids back to fully functioning, no longer avoiding settings, and no longer fearing intense panic attacks. They may continue to have times where they feel low-level, mild symptoms of anxiety and panic, but rather than reacting with fear they manage them and go about their day.

If purposely bringing on panic feelings seems like a poor fit for your child, if your child has medical or physical issues that might interfere with vigorous physical exposures, or if your efforts to do panic exposures are not helping, then it's time to seek out further professional support to guide you and your child through appropriate treatment.

# 14

# Exposure Therapy for Obsessive Compulsive Disorder

When children have obsessive compulsive disorder (OCD) they have two related sets of symptoms. First, they experience intrusive thoughts or urges that make them distressed—obsessions. They then do a repetitive action or ritual to get rid of the distress—compulsions.

Within these patterns of distress followed by ritual, there is a wide range of thoughts, feelings, urges, and actions that can be included in OCD. Many times, the obsessive, intrusive thoughts make kids feel scared or nervous, like maybe germs will make them get sick and die or they will be responsible for something horrible happening. In response, their compulsive hand-washing or other repetitive behavior feels like the only way to keep things safe. Other times, the obsessive thoughts make kids feel disgusted or have the sense that things don't feel right, and the compulsions must be completed until they feel clean or an undefinable balance has been restored. In either case, whether kids feel anxious, disgusted, or just-not-right, exposure is the best treatment.

If we circle back to 14-year-old Hector, you'll remember he has experienced a variety of OCD symptoms since he first began excessive hand-washing in second grade. Currently, his most distressing obsession is that he has thoughts that he wants to stab someone, especially if he is pointing a body part, like his knee, at them. These fears lead to constant monitoring as to how he is holding his body as well as other repetitive rituals to get rid of various upsetting thoughts. In this chapter we will see how Hector and his mother can use exposure to weaken the grip of OCD on his life.

Before beginning exposure therapy to break the cycle of intrusive thoughts and repetitive behavior, it is important to make sure that OCD is the most accurate description for what your child is experiencing, rather than a sign of another issue or condition. This is particularly true when kids are having intrusive thoughts about doing something inappropriate, like hurting themselves or someone else. The key to OCD is that the thoughts don't match how the child is feeling at the moment.

Hector may be in a fine mood, not particularly mad, not particularly happy. He goes into the kitchen where his mother is making breakfast and sees a knife. All of a sudden, he has the thought that he wants to stab his mother, a thought so upsetting that he immediately tries to leave the kitchen, but he can't until he walks through the doorway while having the safe thought that he loves his mother. Contrast that with another 14-year-old boy, Tommy, who, in the middle of an argument with his mother, grabs a knife and threatens to stab her. Grabbing a knife in anger is not OCD, because the thought and its related action, grabbing the knife, are consistent with an emotion: anger. For Hector, the thought of grabbing the knife and hurting his mother has nothing to do with his fine mood that morning, and in fact he fears having such violent thoughts so much that he takes steps to make sure he wouldn't act on them.

Another point to recap here from earlier is that people with OCD do rituals on purpose, but they do not enjoy doing them. Instead, they feel that they have to do them to fix things or feel all right. So, if your child enjoys repetitive behavior, it might not be OCD but rather a preference to be tidy or a self-soothing behavior. In addition, if your child does not realize they are doing a repetitive behavior or if it happens automatically outside their control, it might be a tic rather than OCD. If you are unsure, sometimes going through the avoidance cycle can help sort these issues out.

## STEP 1: BUILDING FROM THE OCD AVOIDANCE CYCLE

A successful exposure plan needs to be individually tailored to your child's needs, starting with your child's avoidance cycle.

### What sets off OCD

First, we need to identify what sets off your child's OCD. Since there are many different variations of OCD, your child's avoidance cycle might be set off by situations, objects, thoughts, or actions. The most familiar type of OCD is set off by contact with objects that might contain germs, such as doorknobs, hand railings, drinking fountains, desks at school, silverware, elevator buttons, public bathrooms, trash cans, or anything and everything that could have been touched by other people or is gross for any other reason. Conversely, OCD can be set off by touching items that your child views as clean, such as their pillow or smartphone. This can happen when your child considers themselves to be already contaminated and wants to keep other things clean.

The OCD avoidance cycle can also be set off by thoughts. Common intrusive thoughts that set off OCD include thoughts about harming oneself or others, being responsible for something bad happening, touching someone inappropriately, or uttering blasphemy. Although these thoughts can be the primary cause of anxiety, because they are upsetting no matter when or where they occur, they may occur more frequently in certain situations, such as seeing a knife in the kitchen, being around children, being in church, or when doing an action, like walking through a doorway. Hector is always upset when he has the thought that he wants to stab someone, but he is more likely to have that thought when he sees a knife, and that thought causes particular problems when he has the thought while leaving a room and has to offset the thought by walking through the doorway while thinking a certain "safe" thought.

OCD can also be set off by actions. When kids experience "just-not-right" OCD, their discomfort may be set off by an action such as putting down a drinking glass, tying one shoe tighter than the other, or touching a wall with only their left hand. Each of these actions sets off the feeling that things are not right, uneven, out of balance. This type of OCD experience can also be set off by seeing objects out of their preferred order, such as items on their desk, the contents of a backpack, or apps left open on a phone.

Frequently though, the OCD avoidance cycle is set off by a combination of thoughts, activities, objects, and situations.

## Expectations that make OCD thoughts and situations upsetting

Once you've identified the situations that set off your child's OCD, the next task is to pinpoint the expectations that cause your child to feel more nervous in these situations than other kids. Just as with other anxiety disorders, the items that set off OCD are safe and ordinary but are upsetting to kids experiencing OCD because they expect something bad will happen or that they won't be able to handle the situation. The most recognizable form of OCD, fear of germs, provides an excellent example of both expectations.

Many kids with OCD fear germs because they think getting germs on their hands or body will lead to something bad happening. A typical contamination expectation would be a statement like this: *If I touch this door handle, the germs will make me get sick and die.*

Other kids with OCD don't think they will get sick; instead the idea of contamination by germs or touching something perceived to be dirty is simply intolerable. A child with this expectation may say something like: *If I touch my shoe it will be so gross and I will never feel comfortable until I get the grossness off my fingers.* Other times, kids are less concerned about themselves and more concerned about spreading germs. They might say something like: *If I get these germs from school on my stuff at home, everything will be ruined and gross.*

Similarly, intrusive thoughts can be scary because kids believe that something bad will happen. They might fear that they will act on a thought: *If I have this thought that I could stab my mother, it must mean that I want to or that I will.* Or they fear that their thoughts will come true. *If I think "Mom will get sick" as I stand up, it will probably happen unless I fix it.*

Kids with OCD also sometimes believe that having certain thoughts makes them a bad person: *If I have thoughts about hurting younger kids, I must be a bad person because a normal good person wouldn't have a thought like this.*

Kids experiencing "just-right OCD" often believe that the discomfort from things being wrong or uneven will build and build and never go away. They might say, *If I only touch something with my right hand I will just feel more and more uneven* or *If I don't tap the cup on the table again it will bother me all day.* Finally, some kids believe that they just can't handle not knowing for sure. If a child's fear is set off by the thought that they might not have locked a door, their expectation may be, *It will be my fault if someone breaks in, and I can't handle not knowing whether the door is locked.*

## Avoidance in OCD

Next, we need to identify the rituals and other avoidance that prevent your child from learning that OCD fears and distress are manageable. OCD is primarily known for avoidance through compulsions that usually involve doing an action over and over again to prevent a feared outcome or to undo something that feels wrong if not corrected.

When kids with contamination-based OCD touch a public surface and they have the thought that they've got germs on their hands now, they respond to the distress by washing their hands more often and thoroughly than they need to. Other compulsions can be repeating an action until it feels right, like picking up and putting a cup down over and over again or touching a wall with their right hand to even things out or always chewing food an even number of times because odd numbers feel unlucky. Rituals may also include checking over and over that doors are locked; turning light switches on and off repeatedly to be sure the lights are off; or checking their smartphone repeatedly to ensure that all apps are closed. Sometimes rituals can be completed silently in the mind only, such as repeating words or saying prayers to undo negative intrusive thoughts. What all these rituals have in common is that something has happened, a thought or contact with contamination, that has made kids feel like something bad or intolerable will happen, and that only by repeating the ritual can they fix things and prevent the bad outcome.

Children who are experiencing OCD may also use physical avoidance of activities and situations to prevent their OCD anxiety. Kids afraid of germs may try to avoid touching public surfaces, for example, using their shoe to push open a door or pulling their sleeve over their hand to tap an elevator button. Hector might avoid going in the kitchen or ask that the sharp knives be put up someplace high out of reach in a cupboard. Other kids may avoid watching shows or movies that have storylines that set off their intrusive thoughts.

Finally, avoidance may also take the form of relying on others, including reassurance seeking. Kids with intrusive thoughts may frequently confess them to their parents. They may tell their parents they had an intrusive sexual thought about a girl they saw at the mall, *Mom, does that mean I'm a terrible person if I had this thought?* Or Hector might ask his father: *Dad, I didn't try to grab the knife, did I?* Relying on others can also include having a parent wash their hands too, clean surfaces excessively with disinfectant wipes, or do extra loads of laundry to clean clothes believed to be contaminated. Parents might also be asked to check locks or avoid entering their child's room so as not to contaminate it.

In the moment, each of these forms of avoidance—physical distance, compulsions, and relying on others—provides relief from the feared outcome, doubts, or distress. However, the relief is short-lived, and when the obsessions occur again, kids feel as if they have no other option than to repeat the rituals. Over time, kids become trapped in the cycle and never have a chance to learn that the distress associated with the thoughts would diminish even if they did not carry out the compulsion.

## STEP 2: BUILDING OCD FEAR LADDERS

Given the variety of objects, thoughts, and activities that set off OCD, there are a number of different types of fear ladders you may need for OCD. Fear ladders for contamination fears are pretty straightforward. The goal is for a child with OCD to be able to handle touching items that they fear are contaminated without having to do their compulsions.

You can start a fear ladder for contamination with an item that seems only slightly contaminated—something that the child or teen would rather not touch but can handle touching without an overwhelming urge to wash their hands. After that first exposure, each step up the fear ladder progresses to items that are more and more contaminated, up to the final exposure, which will include contact with the most contaminated object.

When making a fear ladder for contamination, it's important to remember that we will never do an exposure to things that are dangerous or carry an increased likelihood of getting your child seriously sick. For example, if a child was afraid of getting poisoned from eating food past its expiration date, we would not have them drink spoiled, curdled milk. We only ever do exposures to things that hold the low level of risk that exists in everyday life. So, we may do an exposure to drinking milk that smells okay even if it is a couple days past its sell-by date, as we may do if we forgot to buy milk and need to pour some over cereal on a busy morning.

We do, however, frequently create exposures that see kids more directly and explicitly contaminate themselves than would likely happen in everyday life. For instance, a child might touch a public door handle fully with both hands, then rub her hands together, and then rub her hands on her body and face to spread those door handle germs all over herself. Or toward the end of his fear ladder another child might touch the floor and toilet seat in a public bathroom and then rub the germs all over his clothes, head, and face. Most people think both of those activities are disgusting and wonder why this could possibly be an appropriate exposure. The answer is that while hand-washing is good hygiene, the sequence of events of someone using a public bathroom, dropping something, and touching the floor as they pick it up, then not washing their hands and then shortly after eating a snack occurs frequently in everyday life, even if nobody wants to admit it. We are simply making the connection with contamination more visible in order to more clearly learn that contamination is not as dangerous as your child thinks it is.

Here's an example of a fear ladder for contamination that you can use to get started. The actual items on the list will need to match what your child believes is contaminated.

### Contamination fear ladder

1. Touch a table or chair at home, then rub your hands on your body and don't wash after
2. Touch a doorknob, chair, or railing in a public place, then rub your hands on your body and don't wash after
3. Touch the floor in a public place, then rub your hands on your body and don't wash after
4. Eat after touching something you feel is dirty
5. Touch dirty dishes or silverware, then rub your hands on your body and don't wash after
6. Touch a bathroom sink faucet, then rub your hands on your body and don't wash after
7. Touch a garbage can, then rub your hands on your body and don't wash after
8. Touch a toilet seat in a bathroom at home, then rub your hands on your body and don't wash after
9. Touch the floor in a bathroom, then rub your hands on your body and don't wash after
10. Touch a public toilet flush handle, then rub your hands on your body and don't wash after

For OCD symptoms set off by intrusive thoughts, fear ladders typically involve a list of different thoughts that set off anxiety, combined with items and situations that make it more likely your child will have that thought. The exposures on this fear ladder will be thought, or imaginal, exposures during which your child repeats the upsetting intrusive OCD thought over and over again.

The more challenging exposures will combine repeating the thought in a place, or looking at an object, or doing an activity that makes the thought even more anxiety-provoking. Hector might begin by doing an exposure to repeating the thought *I may stab my mother* while sitting with his father. He then might progress to a more upsetting thought, such as *I want to stab my mother* or *I will stab my mother.* The next steps might include repeating these thoughts while sitting with his mother and holding a knife. It is important for Hector to do exposures where he repeats the exact thoughts that bother him, regardless of how upsetting they are, without adding anything to the thoughts to make exposures easier. If he repeats *I am thinking of stabbing my mother, but I know I never would,* this won't teach him that he can handle upsetting thoughts and is a form of avoidance that he should not engage in.

If your child has one predominant intrusive thought, then the fear ladder can focus on exposures to that thought in more and more challenging ways. When a child has multiple intrusive thoughts, the fear ladder may start off as a list of those intrusive thoughts in order of least to most distressing. It can then have steps to repeat each thought on its own, then in a mildly challenging situation, and then in the most challenging situation.

Another example might include working on compulsive checking in response to fears that the family house might burn down if the child has left the lights on. The first exposure might include repeating the thought: *The house will burn down because I left the lights on.* The next steps could then include repeating this thought after leaving a room with the lights on or after leaving the house without checking the light switch.

Here is a template of the steps you could put on a fear ladder to work on intrusive thoughts.

### Intrusive thoughts fear ladder

1. With a support person (e.g., a parent or therapist), repeat your least upsetting thought over and over
2. Repeat your least upsetting thought over and over alone
3. Repeat a medium upsetting thought over and over
4. Repeat a challenging thought over and over
5. Repeat your most challenging thought over and over
6. Do an activity that makes you worry something bad will happen and repeat that thought over and over
7. Do an activity that makes you worry your worst fear will happen and repeat that thought over and over
8. Tell a trusted person your least upsetting thought
9. Tell a trusted person your most challenging thought

Finally, sometimes we need to build a fear ladder to work on just-right OCD symptoms, where there's not a specific thought, fear, or worry about something bad happening but rather a feeling of things being imbalanced, uneven, or out of order.

Exposures on this type of fear ladder generally involve taking an action or doing something to bring on the not-just-right feeling and sitting with that feeling until the distress goes away without fixing it through a ritual. Sometimes, we can add a thought exposure, such as your child repeating: *This doesn't feel right* or *I will never fix this.*

Often, it is helpful to begin by listing all the compulsions your child does, including the activities they have to do a certain number of times or in a certain way. Then put them in order, beginning with ones that would be easier to do wrong and working up to the ones that are most challenging or upsetting if not done just right. When kids have a very long list of rituals, you can simplify or shorten the list by combining similar rituals. So, if your child taps cups on the table, pencils on her desk, or her phone on the counter, all of these actions fit into the category of tapping things until it feels right.

Here is a sample fear ladder with some activities for working on just-right OCD.

### Just-right fear ladder

1. Mess up your papers or books
2. Leave apps or windows open on your phone or computer
3. Write using imperfect handwriting
4. Read imperfectly
5. Put something down "wrong" without repeating
6. Say or write the word "left" or "right" without saying the other word
7. Touch something with the right (or left) side of your body without touching it with the other side
8. Tap something an odd (or even, if even feels wrong) number of times
9. Step on cracks in the floor
10. Do things the "wrong" number of times
11. Purposely perform routines in the "wrong" order

These three separate fear ladders cover how to plan exposures for the most common forms of OCD: contamination, intrusive thoughts, and just-right rituals. Each of them will need to be tweaked to match the items that set off your child's OCD. However, together they provide a good overview of how to include exposures that involve touching feared surfaces, repeating intrusive thoughts, and bringing on not-just-right feelings.

## STEP 3: SETTING UP OCD EXPOSURES

As with traditional anxiety disorders, exposures for OCD need to be set up as experiments to test the expectations that make ordinary activities distressing. With some exposures, kids are testing the expectation that something bad will happen, expectations like: *The germs will make me sick, I will act on my thought and stab my mother, My dad will get sick if I close the door while thinking he has cancer,* or *I will be punished for thinking I don't believe in God.* Other exposures are experiments to test whether the OCD distress will continue forever unless the child does a ritual, such as *I will feel gross and not be able to use my hand unless I wash,* or *I can't handle not knowing for sure if I turned off the lights,* or *It will bother me all day if I don't even things out.*

Disproving these expectations requires that kids don't do any rituals to fix things. The OCD avoidance cycle continues and worsens because each time kids do a ritual, it strengthens their belief that rituals are necessary to be safe and feel comfortable. So, when choosing an item from the fear ladder for an exposure, it is important for kids and parents to be clear and agree that the child won't do any ritual during *or after* the exposure. If kids know they can wash their hands as soon as the exposure is over, they can often tolerate very high distress because they know it is only temporary until they fix it. So, taking small steps requires picking an exposure that is easy enough that your child feels confident they can handle it without rituals.

## STEP 4: DOING OCD EXPOSURES

When doing exposures for OCD, kids need to stick with an activity long enough and pay attention to what is happening to learn that it is not as dangerous or overwhelming as they had expected. With contamination exposures that generally means having your child touch a contaminated object, rubbing the germs all over their body, and then sitting and thinking about being covered in germs until the distress goes down and the urge to wash passes.

We can increase the focus on anxiety by adding in a thought exposure, such as having kids repeat *These germs will make me and everyone in my family sick* while touching a doorknob. During contamination exposures, you can keep your child focused by periodically gathering anxiety ratings. You can ask *How nervous are you to keep doing this?* or simply *How nervous are you now?* at whatever pace feels frequent enough to catch any changes in distress, but not so often that the ratings are intrusive.

While an initial exposure would likely involve touching one door handle and waiting for anxiety to decrease, a more advanced exposure might include walking around in public and touching many different surfaces. In that case, you might ask *How nervous are you to touch the next doorknob?* after each repetition. When kids are less afraid of getting sick from germs but rather feel disgusted by the idea of contamination, you can rephrase inquiries accordingly and instead ask check-in questions like: *How uncomfortable (or grossed out or upset) are you now?*

You can take a similar approach with thought exposures. As your child repeats the thought over and over, you can check in periodically by asking questions like: *How nervous are you to keep doing this?* or *How nervous are you now?*

As with contamination exposures, if a thought exposure includes doing an action without a ritual, the action is often only done once, and then your child sits with the anxiety while they repeat their thought. A child might walk through a doorway once with the thought *Dad has cancer* and then sit and repeat something like *Dad is going to die of cancer.* Or a child might go to bed without checking that the door is locked or leave the house deliberately with an iPad plugged into the charger. With these types of exposures it is difficult to make the action repetitive for the simple reason that leaving the house to run an errand and coming back over and over is going to be impractical to do multiple times in an afternoon. So, repetition comes in via their saying the thought over and over, such as *Someone will break in because I left the door unlocked* or *The charger will catch fire and burn down the house.*

Finally, exposures for just-right OCD often involve purposely doing actions wrong that will ignite the feeling that it's not been done right and needs to be done as many times as necessary until it feels just right. This can be putting a drinking glass down in a way that feels wrong and then sitting there staring at it, repeating a thought such as *This is wrong, this doesn't feel right* until the urge to fix it passes. It is possible to make this exposure repetitive by picking the glass up only after the urge to fix it has passed and then putting it down deliberately wrong again someplace else and sitting out that feeling to fix it again. Since the compulsion is usually to pick the glass up and put it down multiple times until it feels right, repeating the exposure can be a little too close to ritualizing. For this reason, the exposure is frequently done once, with repetition coming through repeating the thought that this is not just right.

During OCD exposure, you should be attentive to any rituals or other avoidance by your child. If you suspect that your child might be avoiding, you can gently say something along the lines of: *That looks like it might be a ritual to get the germs off your hands?* or *Are you avoiding saying the most upsetting part of this thought?* or *Is that hand movement a ritual?* If your child acknowledges that it was a ritual, no problem, simply have them retouch the germs, or repeat the most difficult thought, or do the action wrong to bring back the OCD discomfort. If they deny it was a ritual, you can say: *Okay, but just to be safe, please don't do that during the exposure.* And then have them redo the action to bring back the OCD discomfort. Be sure to handle this in a warm, supportive, and patient manner.

## STEP 5: ENDING AN OCD EXPOSURE

Each exposure for OCD needs to continue until kids learn they can handle the activity, or thought, or combination of activities and thoughts, without ritualizing. Frequently the foundation of this learning is the decrease in anxiety, disgust, or other distress. When kids expect they will feel gross until they wash, bothered by an uneven feeling, or unable to handle not knowing if the light was off, the decrease in distress teaches them that they did not have to wash their hands, tap the wall with their left hand, or recheck the light switch to feel okay.

This decrease in distress is also important when kids fear something bad will happen. Sometimes, kids' fears can be directly disproven during an exposure. If Hector sits next to his mother holding a knife, repeating *I am going to stab my mother* and nothing happens, he can see he didn't stab his mom. If a child rubs bathroom germs all over himself and nothing happens and he doesn't start feeling sick, the outcome speaks for itself.

However, many OCD worries are future-oriented and won't necessarily occur in the moment. Your child may say, *The bathroom germs won't make me sick right now, it may take a couple days.* Or if they repeat the thought *Dad has cancer* over and over while Dad is at work, your child may say that they can't know whether he is okay unless he has a doctor's appointment and undergoes multiple tests.

Fortunately, exposures can work even if the feared outcome might happen in the future. As a child's anxiety or distress decreases during the exposure through repetition, the chances of something bad happening in the future begin to seem less likely. Kids gradually begin to feel more confident that they can handle not knowing with 100% certainty that everything will be fine.

Sometimes it can help to specifically review these ideas with kids when wrapping up an exposure. If you ask *Did your fear come true?* and your child answers *I won't know until later,* you can follow up with *Is there any evidence right now that your fear is going to come true?* to help them focus on the fact that nothing bad is happening now. And then you can add: *Can you handle not knowing for sure if your fear will come true?* to encourage them to reflect on the fact that they don't need a guarantee of safety—which is never possible anyway in life—to feel okay.

## STEPS 6 AND 7: REPETITION AND WORKING IN THE MOMENT WITH OCD

The basic principles of repetition and building up to on-the-fly exposures apply to OCD as much as the other anxiety disorders. Kids often need to do each exposure more than once before they have it mastered. And the goal of planned exposures is to be able to handle similar situations when they happen in daily life. OCD is unique in the added emphasis we need to put on helping kids to stop doing rituals, which is often called response prevention. This means that after learning through planned exposures that they can handle distress without washing, checking, tapping, evening out, or other rituals, they then need to stop doing those rituals during daily life.

Just like with exposures, we approach response prevention in small steps. We don't expect kids to be able to stop doing all rituals to all feared situations at once. But rather, after kids have learned through planned exposures that they can handle one situation, like door handles, we now expect them to use door handles without washing. But if they come across something harder that we haven't worked on yet, say touching the floor in the hallway, we understand that they may not yet be ready to handle that without washing. The same idea applies to other rituals, such as checking or evening things out.

But how should kids react if they do a ritual? This is a particularly important question when working on contamination fears, where kids are going to wash their hands at normal times during the day, such as after using the bathroom. This is where something we call recontamination comes in. Recontamination is simply getting your hands dirty again after washing. It might mean using the same source of germs. If a child is doing a doorknob exposure and they slip up and use hand sanitizer, that's okay, they can just recontaminate by touching the doorknob again. Or recontamination may involve using a lower-level source of contamination. If this same child washes his hands during the day because he touched a trash can, he might recontaminate his hands by touching a doorknob, because he hasn't done exposure to trash cans yet. The goal is that after finishing exposure to an object such as a doorknob, your child will always have at least some doorknob contamination on their hands.

Although the term *recontaminate* doesn't literally make sense with just-right sensations or intrusive thoughts, the same concept applies. If a child slips up and does a ritual to something we now expect them to handle, they can undo it by making things uneven again, or messing up the order, or repeating a scary thought while walking through a different doorway.

## PARENTS' ROLE WHEN WORKING ON OCD

In addition to coaching your child through planned exposures, you are going to play an important role in making sure your child applies what they learn in daily life. Even after kids have learned that their anxiety will decrease despite not washing the germs off their hands, it's often easier in the moment just to wash and get it over with. This is even more true when rituals can be completed mentally or by quickly tapping the right number of times in the right balance. At those times, a warm but firm reminder that this is a chance to resist rituals and do an on-the-fly exposure can be helpful. Finally, between touching contaminated things and repeating upsetting thoughts, OCD exposures can seem even stranger than exposures for other fears and worries. Kids often need parental support to understand and design exposures that directly challenge their fears.

## COMMON CHALLENGES WITH OCD

One challenge to exposure therapy for OCD is accurately and confidently identifying OCD as the correct understanding of a child's experience. In addition to the example of thoughts involving harming others, self-harming thoughts can be difficult to categorize. While thought exposures are the appropriate treatment for intrusive OCD thoughts that involve hurting oneself, they could be harmful for a child who is feeling suicidal. A teenager with OCD could have intrusive thoughts similar to Hector's, except her thoughts are about stabbing herself with a knife. The thoughts follow the same avoidance cycle, in which despite being in a fine mood, seeing a knife in the kitchen sparks the thought she could stab herself, to which she recoils with fear, and confesses to her mother the thoughts she is having to seek reassurance she has never and would never do something like that. Like Hector, treatment would involve repeating those thoughts until she learns that her scary thought is just that: a thought.

By contrast, another teenager could be feeling sad and depressed and has reached a point where she feels life is not worth living. She has the thought that since nothing will ever get better, her only solution is to attempt to kill herself with the first object available to her, in this case a sharp kitchen knife. Not only is her experience not OCD and not appropriate for exposure therapy, she is likely in need of urgent treatment for depression. Although these examples may be clearly different on paper, in the real world, with your own child, confidently cataloging your child's thoughts of harming themselves as OCD or suicidal thinking can be daunting.

Another challenge with exposure therapy for OCD is that the feared thoughts and situations are upsetting to most people. Some contamination exposures are just plain gross. Parents often have their own doubts about whether a given exposure is hygienic or wise. Intrusive thoughts are frequently about disturbing or taboo topics, like sex, violence, or religion: Things we often don't talk about in public, don't particularly want our kids thinking about, and certainly would rather not encourage our child to repeat out loud. However, if your child is plagued by an upsetting thought, we can't undo that and they don't have the option to avoid it, so exposure is the best treatment solution, despite being unpleasant. Similarly, if your child's fear of germs leaves them with red and raw hands from compulsive and excessive hand-washing, exposure, even if a bit disgusting, is, again, the most appropriate treatment.

## TRACKING PROGRESS ON OCD

Identifying with your child that what they are experiencing is OCD is a significant accomplishment and the first step toward success. Likewise, building a fear ladder full of exposures tailored to your child takes thoughtful study of their avoidance cycle and careful planning and is another milestone not to be taken for granted. Once you get started, successfully completing planned exposures in which your child's distress decreases without rituals is an early sign you are on the right track. With OCD, the most visible symptoms are rituals like hand-washing, tapping, rearranging, checking, and redoing mundane actions, and the gradual fading of these compulsions from your child's daily life is an encouraging sign of your child's success.

It turns out that success does not include getting rid of intrusive thoughts, because having those thoughts is a normal part of being human. Research shows that most people have thoughts similar to OCD thoughts—even the really upsetting ones—but the difference is that most of us, when we have those thoughts, shrug them off and let them go, whereas a child with OCD becomes very fearful of them. So, after successful treatment kids will still have unpleasant thoughts, but they will be better able to let them go and live their lives without compulsive interruptions.

If you are having difficulties finding success with any of these steps, from identifying OCD to figuring out an appropriate fear ladder, to finding the confidence to trust your child to the exposure process, take the knowledge you have gained from your experience to date and seek out a therapist specializing in OCD.

# 15

# Exposure Therapy for Specific Phobias

A specific phobia is the fear of a single, specified object, situation, or activity. The list of items that can be the focus of specific phobias is endless and includes heights, the dark, dogs, bugs, bees, snakes, spiders, storms, elevators, escalators, confined spaces, flying, loud sounds, choking, throwing up, blood, needles, doctors, clowns, mascots, buttons, tall buildings, and deep water. Having fears, even irrational ones, is a normal part of life, especially childhood. Everyday fears cross the line to become problematic phobias when they are not only unfounded—fearing something that is safe—but also make life difficult. Fears of storms, needles, heights, bugs, and throwing up are some of the most common specific phobias that we have seen over the years in our clinic.

As we explore the steps to using exposure therapy to address specific phobias, let's return one last time to Michael and his fear of dogs as an example.

## STEP 1: BUILDING FROM THE SPECIFIC PHOBIA AVOIDANCE CYCLE

A successful exposure plan needs to be individually tailored to your child's needs, and that process starts with an understanding of their avoidance cycle.

### What sets off specific phobias?

First, we need to identify what sets off your child's anxiety. Specific phobias are most often set off by a child coming into contact with or being close to the feared item or being in a situation where they believe they might come into contact with that item. If your child has a specific phobia of bees, they may become very upset when they see a bee buzzing around the garden while they are playing hide-and-seek, or they may be too nervous to even go outside in the summer because there might be a bee.

The same applies to needles, where some children become nervous only right at the moment they are about to get a shot, while others' fears are set off by going to see a doctor because they think they might get a shot. For other phobias, the item that sets off the fear is the situation itself, like being on a balcony setting off a fear of heights or being in light rain setting off a fear of storms.

Specific fears can also be set off by activities. The simple act of eating might set off fears of choking or throwing up. The degree of anxiety may be worse depending on the type of food. Stringy meat that is hard to chew could set off particularly intense fears of choking. Hot dogs, which the child ate just before the last time they vomited, might most reliably set off a fear of throwing up.

Finally, physical feelings may also set off specific phobias. A fear of vomiting may be set off by a queasy feeling in one's stomach, rather than eating.

## Expectations that make specific situations scary

Once you've identified the situations that set off your child's fears, the next thing to do is pinpoint the expectations that cause your child to feel more nervous in these situations than other kids. Most expectations that drive specific phobias are fears of being harmed, as in Michael's fear of dogs. Kids often fear that shots will hurt or that bees will sting them. Sometimes kids, especially younger children, can't specify exactly what it is they are afraid will happen, it's just scary. In these cases, their expectation may be best described as: *I can't handle this,* or *I can't do this without my parents,* or *I will be scared or upset unless I get away from this.*

For some phobias, the fear is not of an object, situation, or activity itself, which might actually be bad, but rather of safe situations that the child associates with that upsetting outcome. Nobody likes throwing up, and most of us find it highly unpleasant, so it is reasonable to be upset if you are actually about to throw up. However, what makes a specific phobia of vomiting a problem is that kids expect that safe, everyday situations, like riding in the car or butterflies in their stomach, will make them throw up. So, while we usually talk about their anxiety as a fear of throwing up, what is really going on is that the child is afraid of riding in the car or stomachaches because they think it will make them throw up.

Similarly, a child might be afraid of sharks, but then again, who isn't? The real problem here is that the child is afraid of swimming in the ocean, or maybe even lakes, because they think there will be a shark and they might get bitten. Understanding the situations that set off your child's anxiety and the expectations that make those situations scary helps you to design an accurate exposure plan.

## Avoidance of specific phobias

Next, we need to identify what avoidance strategies your child is using to stay away from the feared situations and, in doing so, how they are missing out on opportunities to learn that these situations are not as bad as they expect.

With specific phobias, avoidance most often takes the form of maintaining physical distance. Michael hurries inside when he sees the neighbor's dog. Other kids run inside or stay inside to avoid bees. Aaron won't take the elevator and makes his family march up 12 floors every time they leave or return to their hotel room while on vacation. Kids who worry about vomiting may avoid eating certain foods or leaving the house right after eating.

When physical avoidance is not possible, children may rely on their parents to manage the situation, and avoidance can look like asking for excessive reassurance, such as your child repeatedly asking you about the weather report in case a tornado is coming. It can also take the form of screaming, crying, and squirming as a last-ditch effort to avoid getting an essential immunization shot.

### STEP 2: BUILDING SPECIFIC PHOBIA FEAR LADDERS

The content of fear ladders for specific phobias varies greatly due to the wide variety of different phobias but, in general, the ladder consists of action exposures that involve getting physically closer and closer to the feared object, as in the example below of Michael and his fear of dogs.

In addition to increasing physical proximity, steps on a fear ladder can become more challenging by increasing independence. One of Michael's early exposure steps could be to pet his neighbor's dog with his mother; subsequent steps could progress to him petting the dog with only the neighbor around and finally to him petting the dog by himself.

#### A fear ladder for a specific phobia of dogs

1. Watch videos of dogs barking
2. Stand outside a room and look in at a small dog

3. Enter a room with a small dog
4. Pet a small dog
5. Play fetch with and feed a treat to a small dog
6. Go to a friend's house and pet their dog
7. Pet and play with a different, bigger dog
8. Pet and play with younger and older dogs
9. Ask a stranger at the park if you can pet their dog
10. Go to a dog park with a parent

For some phobias, the fear ladder will consist of exposures to the setting where a child thinks their fear may come true rather than the feared object itself. So, for the child who is afraid of bees, the fear ladder might include playing outside by the house, then around bushes, then around flowers in the garden, and then around the garden when there are actually bees flying around. As you might already be thinking, you don't have a lot of control over when and where bees will be, so spontaneous on-the-fly exposures when you encounter bees will be particularly important.

A storm phobia presents similar challenges to planning exposures. If your child has a fear of tornadoes, we're not going to do an exposure to running around outside in the middle of a tornado. That would be dangerous and scary for anyone, and besides that, we can't plan to have a tornado. Instead, the fear ladder will consist of exposures to relatively safe objects, situations, and activities that the child fears. Initial exposures might be to things your child can control and do at a planned time, like watching videos, reading stories about tornadoes, or repeating worry thoughts about tornadoes. Later, more challenging exposures may be weather-dependent but still involve activities that are relatively safe and which most kids could handle. These exposures might include watching a storm through a window, playing outside when its cloudy, going for a car ride when it's rainy, or standing out on the front porch during a thunderstorm. Here is a suggested fear ladder for a phobia of storms. Please use commonsense safety with any fear ladder you create for natural phenomena such as storms.

### A fear ladder for a specific phobia of storms

1. Look at pictures of storms
2. Read stories about powerful storms
3. Watch videos of storms
4. Repeat worry thoughts about having a bad storm rather than checking the weather
5. Stand by a window during a storm (if not a tornado and safe to do so)
6. Drive around with a parent during a storm (if safe to do so)
7. Stand outside while it is raining

A similar approach can be used to build fear ladders for other phobias that involve things we can't encounter on demand. If your child has a specific phobia of bears, we could begin the fear ladder with pictures, videos, and stories about bears and then progress to going to places and doing activities that are safe but bring on the child's fear of bears. This could include walking in the woods, going to the zoo, or having a picnic outdoors.

When kids like Aaron have a fear of heights, they often worry about falling from a height. Of course, we would never purposely have someone fall or do something risky for an exposure. Instead, the fear ladder would include exposures to activities around heights, like standing on a balcony, taking an elevator to a high floor, climbing a ladder, or looking over the wall at the top of a parking structure. Here is an example of a fear ladder for a phobia of heights. For all exposures, please ensure basic safety and accompany your child where age-appropriate.

### A fear ladder for a specific phobia of heights

1. Go up an escalator
2. Ride an elevator
3. Stand by the railing on the lower level of an open parking structure
4. Stand by floor-to-ceiling windows on the top floor of a building
5. Ride in a glass-walled elevator
6. Climb a tall ladder (if safe to do so)
7. Stand on a balcony without holding the railing (if safe to do so)
8. Stand by the railing on the top level of a parking structure with hands in pockets (if safe to do so)
9. Climb a high, open lookout tower (if safe to do so)
10. Walk on a safe and well-maintained path along a scenic overlook

Finally, when planning exposures to choking or vomiting, it is not necessary or appropriate to purposely have a child choke or vomit. This goes back to using the avoidance cycle to understand a child's fears. Specific phobias cause problems because kids are avoiding safe situations and activities that they think are dangerous. In the case of choking or vomiting phobias, fear ladders would consist of eating types of foods in ways and situations that most kids can handle but which make your child very nervous. This might include eating quickly, eating with an appropriate number of bites (rather than over-chewing), eating until very full, eating chewy or stringy food that is harder to swallow, eating oily or smelly food that is a little gross, watching a video of someone throwing up, or taking a car ride after eating.

The fear ladders you build for your child will need to be focused on the specific objects, animals, situations, and activities that set off your child's fears. If your child's fears do not fit into any of the sample fear ladders above, you can adapt them to create an individualized series of exposures tailored to your child's needs.

## STEP 3: SETTING UP SPECIFIC PHOBIA EXPOSURES

Specific phobia exposures are generally set up as experiments to test whether or not the animal, object, situation, or activity is actually harmful to the child. Exposures should be set up to test the expectations that *the dog will bite me, a bee will sting me, I will throw up, I will choke, lightning will hit the house, I will get woozy and fall over the railing, the needle will break off in my arm.*

When kids don't have a clear fear or simply expect the situation to be overwhelming, the expectations to test might be something like *I will panic if I have to keep riding an elevator, I will stay just as scared as I am now for as long as I am looking out the top-floor window, I will freak out if I am on the porch while it is raining.*

Whether the child expects that something bad will happen or simply that their anxiety will build and build, we want to set up that expectation as a clear prediction that we can disprove through each exposure.

For exposures that can't be completed on demand, you might set up a plan with your child to do an exposure at the next available opportunity. For example, once you and your child have completed the early exposures to storm videos and repeating thoughts, you might plan that the next time it rains you will go and sit on the porch.

## STEP 4: DOING SPECIFIC PHOBIA EXPOSURES

Doing exposures for specific phobias can be straightforward. The child simply stays in the situation or repeats the activity that provokes their fear until their anxiety decreases. For Michael, this means watching the dog through the doorway or petting the dog until he decides it is not going to bite him. For Aaron, it might be safely standing at the railing or riding the elevator up and down until he gets bored and realizes he doesn't have to escape to feel safe.

For exposures to address fears of vomiting, your child might watch a short video clip of someone vomiting over and over until they realize it is not going to make them throw up. If a video is long or has lots of non-vomiting parts, it is best to watch and rewatch only the 5 or 10 seconds with the activity of interest. Other exposures for vomiting or choking that involve eating might be made repetitive by eating bite after bite or by repeating scary thoughts after eating.

You can keep your child focused by regularly asking our standard check-in question: *How nervous are you to keep doing this?* When their anxiety goes down, you can follow up with: *That's great! What's bringing it down?* To which we guide kids to answer: *I am petting the dog and guess what, Mom, nothing is happening. She just wants to play.*

It is pretty common for anxiety to go up during specific phobia exposures, not because the exposures are not working but because it is so straightforward to make the exposures more challenging in the moment. For example, Michael is doing an exposure to petting the neighbor's dog, and he starts on the other side of the room from the dog at a 5 out of 10 fear level. After a couple of minutes, he moves halfway across the room, closer to the dog. When his mother asks: *How nervous are you now?* Michael replies he's at a 7 because by getting closer to the dog, he is now doing something more challenging.

Making exposures more challenging in the moment can also happen when kids go from one video (of vomiting or storms, for example) to another, more intense video, or take another step closer to the railing or let go of a parent's hand. These are all positive signs of working hard, so any uptick in anxiety should be accompanied by the understanding that this is happening because your child is stepping up the degree of challenge and certainly not a sign that the exposure is not working.

## STEP 5: ENDING A SPECIFIC PHOBIA EXPOSURE

Exposures need to continue until kids have disproven their fear and demonstrated they can handle the exposure activity. So, when we review how the exposure went, you want to emphasize that what they feared did not come true. The dog didn't bite them, they didn't fall over the edge, the elevator didn't get stuck, no bees stung them, they didn't throw up. Also, you want to help your child realize that they were able to feel calmer and confident during the exposure, without escaping.

## STEPS 6 AND 7: REPETITION AND WORKING IN THE MOMENT WITH SPECIFIC PHOBIAS

Kids will likely need to repeat individual exposures more than once before they feel ready to tackle more challenging or realistic situations. It is also important to keep in mind that kids likely need to practice similar exposures in different situations. Just because Michael becomes comfortable with the neighbor's dog doesn't necessarily mean he will be confident at his aunt's house or with bigger or smaller or younger dogs. He may need to repeat the gradual steps he found successful with his neighbor's dog with a few other dogs before he realizes he can handle most dogs. Likewise, a child who no longer feels the need to hide in the basement at home when there is a thunderstorm may become very anxious during a big storm while vacationing at a small cabin on a lake. Accomplishing sufficient repetition in all the related situations can require a good amount of thoughtful planning by parents.

## PARENTS' ROLE WHEN WORKING ON SPECIFIC PHOBIAS

Because specific phobias often, although by no means always, occur in younger children, as a parent you will be heavily involved throughout and be the driver for starting the process, making the fear ladder, doing exposures, and helping kids use what they have learned in the moment. Even when kids are cooperative it can be helpful for you to put together a motivation plan that includes a simple reward system to celebrate successfully completing exposures and progressing up the fear ladder.

## COMMON CHALLENGES WITH SPECIFIC PHOBIAS

Challenges can arise when working on certain specific phobias. In the case of fully addressing a fear of needles, you will probably need to have your child receive a shot or a blood draw, things that should only be done under medical supervision. Needle phobias need the assistance of a specialist, ideally one working closely with the medical team administering the shots. Other complications can arise when phobias interfere with eating, such as fears of choking or vomiting. When kids aren't receiving adequate nutrition or are losing weight, this can make it more difficult for them to manage their emotions, think flexibly, and be successful with exposure. Weight loss and resistance to eating might also be signs that your child is experiencing medical or mental health problems that need professional evaluation.

## TRACKING PROGRESS WITH SPECIFIC PHOBIAS

Since specific phobias are so focused, your goals for success may be as well. You will know you have accomplished what you set out to do when your child's fear is no longer stopping them from doing the activities they need and want to do, whether that's going to the house of a friend who has a dog, riding the elevator to your 12th-floor hotel room, eating a big lunch before rushing back to class, or playing outside in August while bees pollinate the garden. To have succeeded, your child does not have to be free of fear, nor do they have to get the better of their anxiety at every turn; they simply need to live as independently as expected for their age. If despite your best efforts to implement exposures as a family your child continues to struggle with their fears, I recommend that you seek out the help of a therapist.

# Afterword

Going forward, I encourage you to pursue one of two paths. First, if you think exposure is an accurate and doable next step for addressing your child's anxiety or OCD, then please get to work. Share what you have learned with your child, and if they are interested, invite them to read the book as well. There is nothing written here that we wish to hide from kids or want only parents to know. We are all in this together, and we should do everything we can to make sure we are on the same page.

On the other hand, if you remain uncertain about whether exposure is right for your child, or if the problems your child is dealing with are simply more than a family can address alone, then let's find you some further help. What you have learned through this book has hopefully made you a highly informed consumer who knows what to look for to get the best help for your child. To that end, we have included a list of resources near the end of the book to help you find a therapist with expertise in anxiety, OCD, and exposure therapy.

Please remember that anxiety and OCD are treatable. If your first attempt, whether on your own or with a therapist, is not successful, that does not mean the next attempt won't be. Some fears and worries are more stubborn than others, but help is always available.

*Sincerely,*
*Dr. Stephen P. H. Whiteside*

# Acknowledgments

This book would never have been possible without the support, mentoring, teamwork, partnership, love, and patience of more people than I can acknowledge here. With apologies to those I miss, the people most directly responsible include those at Mayo Clinic Press, who gave me the opportunity to write this book; my editor, Daniela Rapp, whose patience with my naivete about how to write a book appears to be limitless; and my co-writer, Nick Johnstone, who somehow worked his magic to make my dry academic writing interesting and readable.

I would never have written this book without decades of clinical experience watching kids get better and research demonstrating that our parent-coached exposure is more effective than the best alternatives. Neither of those achievements would have occurred without the professionalism, dedication, expertise, patience, and hard work of the Pediatric Anxiety Disorders Clinic staff: Dr. Mark Olsen, Dr. Bridget Biggs, Mike Tiede, Julie Dammann, Stephanie Reneson-Feeder, Megan Cunningham, MacKenzie Urban, Matt Brickl, Deanna Hofschulte, Kim Bailey, Andrea Hillson Jensen, and Kay Nevinger. We have learned together, and everything we have accomplished we have accomplished together.

When it comes to what I know about anxiety, OCD, and exposure therapy, it is fair to say I knew nothing until I was taught by Dr. Jonathan Abramowitz. Jon launched me on the path of learning about child anxiety and OCD, and his knowledge and expertise are only surpassed by his generosity as a mentor. I will also always be indebted to Dr. Donald Lynam, who instilled in me the importance of thinking critically and gave me the tools to do the research to answer the resulting questions. And to Dr. Paul Kettlewell, who seemingly effortlessly demonstrated that it is possible to be a clinician and scientist while simultaneously being dedicated to your family and an overall wonderful person day in and day out.

And finally, thanks to my family: My parents and sister, whose unwavering love and support allows me to try anything and fail and try again. My amazing wife, Catherine, whose expertise in exposure therapy acquired over years of patiently listening to me drone on, along with her natural expertise in motherhood, clear and concise communication, and desire for me not to look like a pompous twit made her the world's best proofreader. And to my wonderful daughter, Geneva, who brilliantly sums up my entire professional existence as "He helps kids with anxiety by having them repeat 'I'm gonna die, I'm gonna die, I'm gonna die' until they aren't scared anymore."

To all of these people, and the many more friends, colleagues, and family members, I am grateful for your support and hope that I give as much as I receive.

# Further Resources

One of the greatest and most frustrating challenges when seeking mental health treatment for your child is finding a qualified therapist. Although at this point you are highly knowledgeable about anxiety, OCD, and exposure, no written word can replace the sense of empowerment from a warm, experienced mental health professional. Fortunately, there are organizations working tirelessly to make high-quality therapy more available.

**Association for Behavioral and Cognitive Therapies** (ABCT): ABCT has been my professional home for over 20 years and is the foremost organization promoting the use of behavior therapy to achieve better mental health. Not all therapists who belong to ABCT specialize in anxiety disorder or OCD or work with kids and teenagers, but they are bound by a commitment to treatment designed to help change behavior, including exposure. Their website (www.abct.org) allows you to search for therapists who are in your home area, willing to work with kids, and specialize in anxiety or OCD.

**International OCD Foundation (IOCDF):** I have been a member of IOCDF for over 20 years and am forever grateful to them for the research grants that supported our imaging studies of OCD and exposure therapy. No organization has done more to train therapists in exposure and response prevention for OCD and to support patients and families through their journey living with OCD. If you are looking for a therapist specializing in the most effective treatment for OCD, there is no better source than their website (www.iocdf.org).

**Anxiety and Depression Association of America** (ADAA): ADAA is another professional organization focused on supporting those suffering from anxiety, as well as depression, through education, training, and the dissemination of research. Their website (www.adaa.org) allows you to search for therapists who are in your home area, willing to work with kids, and specialize in anxiety.

## APPENDIX

# Exposure Therapy Worksheet

### STEP 1: BUILDING FROM THE AVOIDANCE CYCLE

A successful exposure plan needs to be individually tailored to your child's needs. And that process starts with an understanding of the avoidance cycle. Answer the questions below to describe your child's avoidance cycle so that you can structure your child's experience in a way that helps start exposure therapy.

**What sets off your child's anxiety or OCD?** Remember, it could include situations and activities, thoughts in your head, feelings in your body, or a combination of these.

_______________________________________________

_______________________________________________

**What does your child expect to happen that makes safe situations scary?** If they are afraid of something bad happening, be specific. If they think they simply won't be able to handle it, describe what they think it will be like for them in this feared situation.

_______________________________________________

_______________________________________________

**How does your child avoid feared situations that prevent them from learning the situations aren't so bad?** Remember, avoidance includes keeping physical distance (partial or complete), performing rituals and over-preparing (like washing hands or studying much longer than needed), or relying on others (like asking you as their parents if everything will be okay).

________________________________________

________________________________________

## STEP 2: BUILDING FEAR LADDERS

Now that you understand how your child's experience fits into an avoidance cycle, let's use that to make a fear ladder. Start with the items you wrote down that set off your child's anxiety or OCD and then make a list of all the ways, places, and times that their fears, worries, or OCD happen.

________________________________________

________________________________________

________________________________________

Now, plan an exposure, or more than one, to work on each of the items that set off their fears, worries, and OCD symptoms. List exposures from easiest to hardest. If your child has more than one source of anxiety, you will need to draw up more than one fear ladder.

### Fear Ladder

1. ____________________________________

2. ____________________________________

3. ____________________

4. ____________________

5. ____________________

6. ____________________

7. ____________________

8. ____________________

9. ____________________

10. ____________________

## STEP 3: SETTING UP A PLANNED EXPOSURE

With your child, pick an item from the fear ladder together. Remember, though we need to move forward, we should take small steps, so the items on the fear ladder don't have to be tackled in order.

We are going to do an exposure to:

____________________

____________________

Now, set this exposure up as an experiment by using the expectations you identified in the avoidance cycle. What is your child afraid is going to happen? If it's something bad, then what? Or do they think they just won't be able to handle being anxious? Have your child complete this sentence:

When I do this exposure, I am afraid that:

Finally, ask your child how nervous they are to do this exposure, where 0 is not at all and 10 is totally terrified:

## STEP 4: DOING EXPOSURES

This is the moment we have been planning for, when you and your child will do an exposure together. Your job, as the exposure coach, is to be warm and supportive and make sure your child stays on track.

As you go, keep an eye out for any avoidance, rituals, or reassurance requests by your child that will stop them from learning that the feared situation is actually reasonably safe.

Ask your child every couple of minutes, "How nervous are you to keep doing this?" and record their numerical answers (0 to 10) on the chart below.

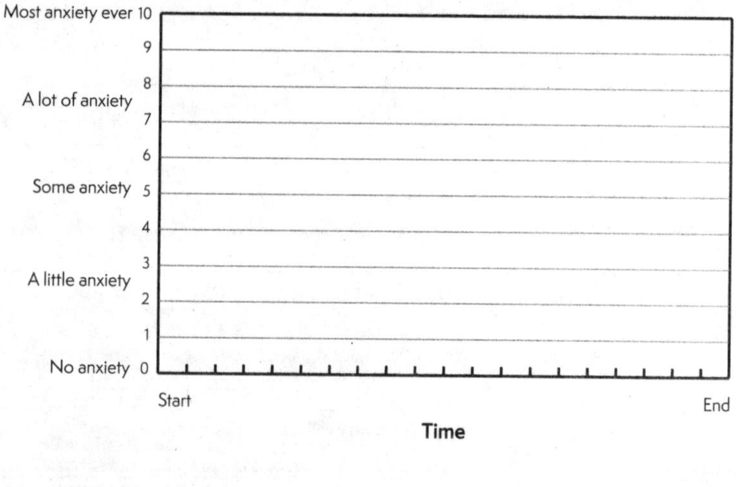

If their anxiety stays high, praise them for working hard and managing their emotions. When their anxiety comes down, ask them: "What's bringing your anxiety down?" Ideally your child will reply: "I am facing my fears and nothing bad is happening!"

## STEP 5: ENDING AN EXPOSURE

Stick with each exposure until your child can say: "That's not so bad, I could do that again!" Usually that means that their anxiety has come down by half. Before you are done, make sure your child has learned from the exposure by having them answer these two questions:

### Did your fear come true?

_______ No

_______ Yes, but it wasn't bad

_______ Other (something's not right, we need to see what happened)

### What happened to your anxiety?

_______ It went down

_______ It stayed high, but I handled it

_______ Other (something's not right, we need to see what happened)

## STEPS 6 AND 7: REPETITION AND WORKING IN THE MOMENT

As your child gradually relearns to feel safe, exposures need to be repeated over and over in all the different real-life daily situations in which fear, worries, and OCD bother them. Each time they do an exposure to an item on the fear ladder, put a checkmark next to that item to show their progress. After you have done a few planned exposures, you can start adding in some on-the-fly exposures. Once you feel that your child has mastered an item from the fear ladder, cross it off.

## PARENTS' ROLE

Your role is to be a warm and supportive hands-on exposure coach who leads your child through planned exposures and then encourages their independence as they transition to on-the-fly exposures in everyday life.

Here are some questions that will help you set goals and make a motivation plan:

My child and I plan to do this many exposures each week:

____________________________________________________________

____________________________________________________________

After we have completed ______ exposures we will celebrate with this prize or fun activity:

____________________________________________________________

____________________________________________________________

If my child refuses to do an exposure, they will lose the following privileges until it is done:

____________________________________________________________

____________________________________________________________

## COMMON CHALLENGES

Like most things, exposure therapy rarely goes totally smoothly. Keep a list of challenges and bumps along the way. If you find that you are not making progress, you can share this list with a therapist or mental health professional for help getting unstuck.

______________________________________________

______________________________________________

## TRACKING PROGRESS

Exposure therapy for anxiety and OCD takes time to be effective. Some improvements happen gradually and are easy to overlook. Use this checklist to track your child's progress:

_______ Completed the avoidance cycle

_______ Built one or more fear ladders

_______ Did a practice exposure and discussed the general idea of what we're going to do

_______ Completed a successful exposure where my child felt nervous at first but stuck with it until they felt better

_______ Started doing some on-the-fly exposures

_______ Checked some items off the fear ladder because my child has mastered them

_______ Planned a mastery exposure

_______ Completed a mastery exposure

## MOVING ON

You will know it's time to move on from exposure therapy when fear, worry, or OCD are no longer interfering with your child's life. Your child still gets anxious and upset sometimes, but it doesn't stop them from participating in school, hanging out with friends, and taking part in family activities. Your child should also appear to be calmer, more confident, and less worried and nervous than before.

# Index